T0231397

FINAL FRCR PART A
MODULES 1–3
SINGLE BEST ANSWER MCQs

FINAL FRCR PART A
MODULES 1–3
SINGLE BEST ANSWER MCQs

THE SRT COLLECTION OF 600 QUESTIONS WITH EXPLANATORY ANSWERS

Edited by

ROBIN PROCTOR
MA (Cantab) FRCR MRCP MRCGP
Specialist Registrar in Clinical Radiology
Southampton General Hospital
President, Society of Radiologists in Training

Foreword by

JOANNA FAIRHURST
Head of Training
Wessex Radiology Training Scheme
Consultant Paediatric Radiologist
Southampton University Hospitals Trust

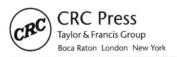

CRC Press
Taylor & Francis Group
Boca Raton London New York

CRC Press is an imprint of the
Taylor & Francis Group, an **informa** business

Radcliffe Publishing Ltd
18 Marcham Road
Abingdon
Oxon OX14 1AA
United Kingdom

www.radcliffe-oxford.com
Electronic catalogue and worldwide online ordering facility.

© 2009 The Society of Radiologists in Training

The Society of Radiologists in Training has asserted its right under the Copyright, Designs and Patents Act 1998 to be identified as the author of this work.

All rights reserved. No part of this publication may be reproduced, stored in a retrieval system or transmitted, in any form or by any means, electronic, mechanical, photocopying, recording or otherwise, without the prior permission of the copyright owner.

British Library Cataloguing in Publication Data

A catalogue record for this book is available from the British Library.

ISBN-13: 978 184619 363 7

The paper used for the text pages of this book is FSC certified. FSC (The Forest Stewardship Council) is an international network to promote responsible management of the world's forests.

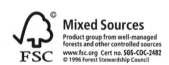

Mixed Sources
Product group from well-managed
forests and other controlled sources
www.fsc.org Cert no. SGS-COC-2482
© 1996 Forest Stewardship Council

Typeset by Pindar NZ, Auckland, New Zealand

Contents

Foreword

It is never easy to decide how best to prepare for an examination: should one concentrate on reading detailed textbooks in the hope that a sufficient proportion of the facts are retained? Are books written as examination aides enough? Should a candidate peruse the recent literature in case 'hot topics' are covered in the questions? Or in this age of increasing reliance on electronic information, should the candidate place their hopes in electronic teaching files? Whatever their personal preference, it is likely that most candidates will turn to examples of examination questions in order to help gauge their preparedness for a test and assess their progress in acquiring the necessary knowledge. The number of publications available to radiologists in training to help them prepare for the Part 2A examination for the FRCR is an indication of how popular these books are as an examination aide. Over the years these texts have been able to draw on the recollections of questions encountered by past candidates and on the expertise acquired by question-setters from a variety of backgrounds. Neither of these resources is available to the candidate about to sit the new single best answer format that the Royal College of Radiologists has adopted for the new-style 2A examination modules. This style of question has been used successfully in the medical world for a number of years, but is novel and unexplored in the context of the FRCR.

Thankfully the authors of this book have responded to the challenge of producing a volume that can provide candidates with experience of attempting to answer questions in this new format. They have collaborated to develop a large number of questions in the new style and have organised these into papers along the lines of the six 2A modules, to give readers the best chance of reproducing the feel of the new examination before sitting the real thing. This has indeed been a significant challenge: not only have the authors had to develop their own question-writing skills along new lines, but they have also had to judge how the full core curriculum will be assessed in this new format and how to therefore organise the papers to reflect likely examination topics. As a past Examiner I can testify to the difficulty in preparing questions that are sufficiently rigorous in their factual content, unambiguous in their interpretation and pertinent to the curriculum to be accepted for inclusion in the FRCR 2A exam. The authors have done an admirable job in drawing together a large number of high-quality questions that satisfy these criteria.

I have no doubt that candidates sitting the 2A exam will find this book a vital tool in their preparation. It provides a unique collection of questions that will help familiarise candidates with the new format, and demonstrate how their knowledge will need to be applied to maximise their chance of success when attempting single best answer papers. The authors are well placed to use their up-to-date knowledge of the Fellowship exam to guide future exam hopefuls through the pitfalls of the new format, and this publication should find its way onto many radiologists' bookshelves in the near future.

Joanna Fairhurst
Head of Training
Wessex Radiology Training Scheme
Consultant Paediatric Radiologist
Southampton University Hospitals Trust
June 2009

Preface

This book has been written by a large number of current trainees in Clinical Radiology and has been coordinated through The Society of Radiologists in Training (SRT). The SRT is the only national organisation of Radiology Trainees in the UK and is run by an elected committee to promote radiology training and education. The SRT organises an annual meeting for trainees and hosts an active website: www.thesrt.org.uk

This book is of particular relevance to higher trainees within radiology who are working towards the Final FRCR examination of the Royal College of Radiologists in the UK. This examination is in the process of being revised and single best answer (SBA) type questions will be introduced in Part A for the first time at the Autumn 2009 sitting. This type of question is well established in other professional examinations but there are currently no published texts of such questions in Clinical Radiology so this book will meet a real need and aid candidates in their preparation. Candidates for other professional exams in Radiology will also find the text useful and those from other specialties will be able to explore the radiological aspects of their syllabus in greater depth.

More than 20 contributing authors, who all have very recent memory of sitting the Part A component of the Final FRCR examination, have written over 1250 single best answer questions and explanations covering the whole breadth of Clinical Radiology. As in the actual examination, readers will find that important topics have deliberately been covered by more than one author in more than one style and we hope, in addition to the factual information presented, that this will illustrate our interpretation of the various ways in which this style of question may be phrased.

The questions are grouped by topic and split into three papers of 70 questions each. This is very similar to the Royal College format of 75 questions per paper. The explanations have been separated into separate chapters so that readers may either attempt a whole mock exam paper or browse through question by question. This book is intended as a bridge between a pure revision aid and a reference text and we include a bibliography of useful references for further information. There are also references to a small number of particularly relevant journal articles within the explanations.

We thank the many colleagues who have given their time and experience in helping write the questions and thank Chuks Ihezue for his help with the genito-urinary questions. We wish every candidate success and would always be grateful for feedback, which can be submitted via the Society Website or email: president@thesrt.org.uk

Robin Proctor
June 2009

About the editor

Robin Proctor MA (Cantab) FRCR MRCP MRCGP
Specialist Registrar in Clinical Radiology, Southampton General Hospital

Robin read medicine at Churchill College, Cambridge where he won a college scholarship before completing his clinical studies at Balliol College, Oxford, winning the prize in Orthopaedic Surgery in the process. He subsequently completed MRCP before training as a General Practitioner and being awarded MRCGP with distinction. He then worked as a GP and Police Surgeon until returning to Hospital Medicine in 2005 as a Specialist Registrar in Radiology. He completed FRCR in 2008. He enjoys teaching medicine and has authored a number of books and articles including a randomised trial comparing teaching methods for medical students.

He has also worked as the expedition leader and medical officer on a diving expedition to the Philippines and in his spare time he enjoys the outdoors, teaches sub-aqua diving and particularly enjoys sailing on the west coast of Scotland.

He has been SRT President since 2007 and conceived this project to produce single best answer MCQs for the new Final FRCR Part A examination as part of a strategy to keep the SRT at the forefront of Radiology training.

Contributors

CHAPTER COORDINATORS
Cardiothoracic and vascular radiology
Charlotte E Lane MRCP FRCR
Specialist Registrar in Clinical Radiology, Southampton General Hospital

Charlie qualified from Nottingham University Medical School in 2000 and initially worked in North Yorkshire and Nottingham before moving to Bournemouth to complete a medical rotation. She passed MRCP in 2004 and accepted a place on the Wessex radiology training scheme the same year. She completed the Fellowship examination of the Royal College of Radiologists in October 2008. She has publications in genito-urinary radiology and an active interest in both medical student and postgraduate teaching. Although training as a general radiologist, her subspecialty interests include cardiothoracic, paediatric and women's imaging.

Musculoskeletal and trauma radiology
Dhiren Shah MA (Cantab) MRCS
Specialist Registrar in Clinical Radiology, Guy's and St Thomas' Hospitals

Dhiren Shah read medicine at Robinson College, Cambridge, where he received a college prize and scholarship, and St. George's Hospital, London, graduating with distinction. He completed surgical training in London and Bristol and passed MRCS in 2006.

He has an active interest in teaching and postgraduate education, having tutored medical students as an Anatomy Demonstrator and provided numerous undergraduate and postgraduate radiology tutorials. Dhiren was selected as a trainee partner for the Postgraduate Medical Education and Training Board (PMETB) in 2008. He is regularly invited to PMETB panels and deanery visits to help ensure postgraduate training programmes and curricula continue to meet PMETB objectives, thus helping to safeguard the quality of medical training in the UK.

Noteworthy achievements include the prestigious 'Magna Cum Laude'

Award at the 2008 RSNA Annual Meeting. His subspeciality interests include musculoskeletal, cardiac and interventional radiology.

Gastrointestinal and hepatobiliary radiology
Nick Railton MBBS FRCR
Specialist Registrar in Clinical Radiology, Southampton General Hospital

Nick qualified from Guy's, King's and St Thomas' medical schools in 2000. He was appointed as a vascular research fellow in the department of academic surgery and vascular medicine at King's College Hospital in 2002. In this post he worked as a sub-investigator on a series of multi-centre clinical trials and published several scientific articles. He subsequently completed his basic surgical training at Homerton University Hospital.

He has been working as a radiology registrar at Southampton University Hospital since 2005 and during his specialist training he has developed interests in education and interventional radiology. He is the current Vice-President of the Society of Radiologists in Training and is the junior representative to the educational committee of the British Society of Interventional Radiology. He was recently appointed as the fellow in hepatobiliary and non-vascular intervention at Southampton.

CONTRIBUTING AUTHORS
Cardiothoracic and vascular radiology
Charlotte E Lane MRCP FRCR
Specialist Registrar in Clinical Radiology, Southampton General Hospital

James Shambrook MRCP FRCR
Specialist Registrar in Clinical Radiology, Southampton General Hospital

Joseph Jacoby BSc (Hons) MBBS MRCP
Specialist Registrar in Clinical Radiology, Southampton General Hospital

Shaun Xavier JM Chan MBBS (Melbourne) PGDipECHO (Melbourne)
Specialist Trainee in Clinical Radiology, Singapore General Hospital

Nick Railton MBBS FRCR
Specialist Registrar in Clinical Radiology, Southampton General Hospital

Musculoskeletal and trauma radiology
Dhiren Shah MA (Cantab) MRCS
Specialist Registrar in Clinical Radiology, Guy's and St Thomas' Hospitals

Gregor Stenhouse MRCS
Specialist Trainee in Clinical Radiology, St Mary's Hospital, Imperial College

Jennifer Davidson MBBS BA MRCS
Specialist Trainee in Clinical Radiology, Southampton General Hospital

Gastrointestinal and hepatobiliary radiology
Nick Railton MBBS FRCR
Specialist Registrar in Clinical Radiology, Southampton General Hospital

Sharmila K Rao MBBS BSc (Hons)
Specialist Registrar in Clinical Radiology, Southampton General Hospital

Beth Shepherd MA (Cantab) MBBS MRCS
Specialist Registrar in Clinical Radiology, Southampton General Hospital

Thomas Jones MA (Cantab) MBBS
Specialist Registrar in Clinical Radiology, University Bristol Hospitals NHS Foundation Trust

Nuclear medicine
Sarah Cook MBBS MRCS FRCR
Specialist Registrar in Radiology, Southampton General Hospital

Abbreviations

ACE	angiotensin converting enzyme
AICA	anterior inferior cerebellar artery
AIDS	acquired immune deficiency syndrome
ACL	anterior cruciate ligament (of knee)
ADC	apparent diffusion coefficient map
ALP	alkaline phosphatase
AP	anteroposterior
ASD	atrial septal defect
AVM	arteriovenous malformation
AVSD	atrio-ventricular septal defect
AXR	plain abdominal radiograph
βHCG	beta human chorionic gonadotropin
bpm	beats per minute
BRCA	breast cancer, early onset (tumour suppressor gene)
CC	craniocaudal
CMV	*Cytomegalovirus*
CNS	central nervous system
CPAP	continuous positive airways pressure
CSF	cerebro-spinal fluid
CPR	cardiopulmonary resuscitation
CT	computed tomography
CVA	cerebrovascular accident
CVP	central venous pressure
CXR	chest radiograph
DaTSCAN	dopamine transporter scan
DCIS	ductal carcinoma *in situ*
DDH	developmental dysplasia of the hip
DMSA	tc-99m-dimercaptosuccinic acid
DTPA	tc-99m-diethylenetriamine pentaacetic acid
DVT	deep vein thrombosis
DWI	diffusion weighted imaging
ECA	external carotid artery
ECG	electrocardiogram

ENT	ear, nose and throat
ERCP	endoscopic retrograde cholangio pancreatography
ESR	erythrocyte sedimentation rate
FAST	focused abdominal sonography in trauma
FDG	fluorodeoxyglucose
FESS	functional endoscopic sinus surgery
FEV1	forced expiratory volume in 1 second
FLAIR	fluid attenuated inversion recovery
FNA	fine needle aspirate
FSH	follicle stimulating hormone
FVC	forced vital capacity
GBM	glioblastoma multiforme
GCS	Glasgow Coma Score
GFR	glomerular filtration rate
GOJ	gastro-oesophageal junction
GU	genito-urinary
HIDA	hepatobiliary iminodiacetic acid
HIV	human immunodeficiency virus
HMPAO	hexamethyl-propylene amine oxime
HRCT	high resolution computed tomography
HRT	hormone replacement therapy
HU	Hounsfield units
ICA	internal carotid artery
ICU	intensive care unit
ITU	intensive therapy unit
IUGR	intra-uterine growth retardation
IV	intravenous
IVC	inferior vena cava
IVP	intravenous pyelogram
IVU	intravenous urogram
KUB	X-ray of kidneys, ureters and bladder
LAD	left anterior descending (artery)
LCIS	lobular carcinoma *in situ*
LCL	lateral collateral ligament (of knee)
LDH	lactate dehydrogenase
LVH	left ventricular hypertrophy
LH	luteinising hormone
LOC	loss of consciousness
MAG3	tc-99m-mercaptoacetyltriglycine
MCA	middle cerebral artery
MCL	medial collateral ligament (of knee)
MCUG	micturating cystourethrogram
MCV	mean cell volume
MDP	tc-99m methylene-diphosphonate
MEN	multiple endocrine neoplasia

MHA-TP	microhaemagglutination treponema pollidum test
MIBG	meta-iodobenzylguanidine
MLO	medio-lateral oblique
MRCP	magnetic resonance cholangio pancreatography
MRI	magnetic resonance imaging
MS	multiple sclerosis
MUGA	multi-gated acquisition scan
NAI	non-accidental injury
NF1	neurofibromatosis type 1
NF2	neurofibromatosis type 2
NG	nasogastric
OCP	oral contraceptive pill
OPG	orthopantomogram radiograph
PA	posteroanterior
PCOS	polycystic ovarian syndrome
PD	proton density
PDA	patent ductus arteriosus
PE	pulmonary embolus
PET	positron emission tomography
PICA	posterior inferior cerebellar artery
PID	pelvic inflammatory disease
PNET	primitive neuroectodermal tumour
PPH	post-partum haemorrhage
PSA	prostate specific antigen
PTH	parathyroid hormone
RI	resistance index
ROI	region of interest
RSV	respiratory syncytial virus
RTA	road traffic accident
SCA	superior cerebellar artery
SPECT	single photon emission computed tomography
STIR	short tau inversion recovery
SUV	standardised uptake value
SVC	superior vena cava
T1	T1-weighted MRI
T2	T2-weighted MRI
T2*	T2 'star' weighted MRI
TCC	transitional cell carcinoma
TNM	tumour, nodes and metastases cancer staging system
TSH	thyroid stimulating hormone
US	ultrasound
USS	ultrasound scan
VACTERL	syndrome of vertebral, anal, cardiac, tracheo-oesophageal fistula/oesophageal atresia, renal and limb abnormalities
VDRL	Venereal Disease Research Laboratory test

VF	ventricular fibrillation
V/Q scan	ventilation/perfusion scan
VSD	ventricular septal defect
VUJ	vesicoureteric junction
WCC	white cell count

Introduction

THE NEW FRCR 2A SYLLABUS

The Royal College of Radiologists (www.rcr.ac.uk) sets the FRCR examination and will provide guidance notes and a syllabus to prospective candidates on request. These comments are our current interpretation of what the college intends but candidates should check with the college that they remain applicable.

The Final FRCR Part A syllabus has been revised and some topics have been removed, notably physics and anatomy. These remain important to Clinical Radiology and will be tested elsewhere, but it does not make sense to specifically revise them for the Final FRCR Part A examination in which they are not included. It is likely that some applied knowledge will remain applicable when directly clinically relevant, but pure anatomy and pure physics are no longer scheduled to be included.

The vast majority of the questions will be clinical questions and this is reflected in the content of this book. Do not be misled by the name of the examination modules, particularly the shortened term usually used by candidates, for example, Module 4 is 'GU' or Module 6 'Neuro'. While there will of course be genito-urinary questions in the 'GU' exam there will also be questions on renal, adrenal and breast radiology. Similarly, within the 'Neuro' module there will be questions on the jaw, teeth, eye and ophthalmology conditions, ENT and spinal pathology. While Neuroradiology questions may be the largest single group it may be that they do not even make up a majority of the exam, hence reading the syllabus and targeting exam preparation to all the topics that may be included is important.

There is also a number of general conditions that could appear in any module such as lymphoma, leukaemia, TB, HIV, NAI, melanoma, unknown primary, etc. For instance, it may be that the vignette and stem are based in the core of that module but that the question probes how that condition may extend to involve another organ or system. Consequently, a good general knowledge of such conditions may be useful.

Finally, our interpretation of the syllabus is that questions on statistics could be included and we have incorporated a handful in this book. While they are unlikely to form a large component of the exam it is likely that they will be comparatively easy marks for those who have a basic grasp of medical statistics and we hope the topics we cover will recur in the real exam.

HOW TO APPROACH SINGLE BEST ANSWER QUESTIONS

While these questions may test similar knowledge, they are different from true/false multiple choice questions and require different skills to answer them.

In preparing both these comments and the remainder of the book in general we have studied the published advice from the Royal College regarding the planned change in format of the FRCR examination. We found McCoubrie and McKnight's article in *Clinical Radiology* an extremely useful summary of the process and would recommend it to all prospective candidates for the new FRCR 2A examination. (McCoubrie P, McKnight L. Single best answer MCQs: a new format for the FRCR Part 2a exam. *Clinical Radiology*. 2008; **63**(5): 506–10). For those who wish a more in-depth text we suggest the National Board of Medical Examiners (NBME) Item Writing Manual, which is available for free download from www.nbme.org/PDF/ItemWriting_2003/2003IWGwhole.pdf While this is written for those setting questions (and NBME have been involved in the training of the regional panels who set questions for the RCR) this manual will give candidates a good background of the important issues regarding multiple choice questions of all types in the clinical setting.

Style of question

The new style question will require the candidate to read a 'vignette' – a sentence or paragraph setting the scene, which is likely to be a clinical scenario – and then to read and consider a question before picking the best answer from five possible options. These questions are widely established in other areas of clinical medicine, although they are relatively new to Radiology. They are better suited to testing more applied knowledge and compared to true/false questions it is hoped that performance will depend more on knowledge than technique. Previously, with true/false questions, exam savvy candidates who may be stronger on technique than knowledge may have done much better than expected. Similarly, it will no longer be possible to associate individual words in the question and answer to work out the correct answer and it is likely that a greater command of written English will be required with single best answer questions than with the true/false style. It is also hoped that the knowledge tested will be more applied and there will be less scope for learning (or having to learn) 'just for the exam'.

The ideal question will test how to apply knowledge in a particular scenario and will require both the knowledge itself and the correct application of this knowledge to succeed rather than just the knowledge alone. The aim is for questions in the 'Who wants to be a Millionaire?' format, which can almost always be answered by a good candidate before reading the possible options. (In medical education jargon, no cue is needed from the options.)

In the ideal question all the options should be 'homogeneous' or 'on the same continuum' hence while the correct option should clearly be identifiable (and should be very much more likely than the others) the other options may remain possible but much less likely and are unlikely to all be entirely wrong.

There are a number of options for how to construct good questions and after attempting a number of practice questions candidates will better appreciate how the questions are constructed. Particularly in Clinical Radiology, there is likely to be an initial description giving some combination of the clinical history, pathological, radiological and examination findings. The question part may then ask about the diagnosis, differential treatment, radiological findings (if not already given or in a different modality) or associated features. For most questions the options are likely to be presented as a list, but for some questions, for instance staging lung cancer, tabulating the options works well.

When writing these questions it is possible to put a number of twists in the question or to take the question several levels away from the answer and this application of knowledge can make a question more discriminatory.

Different formats

The intention is usually to examine important information rather than what is easy to test and we suspect that the majority of questions will do this in the SBA format. There are some topics, however, which are particularly difficult to access in the new format and it remains to be seen what the Royal College Examiners will choose to do. It may be that they do not include these topics or find a novel way of approaching the information in SBA format, but we think it more likely that some topics will be examined with questions of a different format and this is the route we have chosen to take in this book where we have opted to vary the format of the questions slightly for these few topics to include particularly important information that we feel is likely to be incorporated in the College examinations.

The ideal SBA question will not be phrased in the negative and use terms such as NOT, LEAST LIKELY or EXCEPT. For some of the topics that are difficult to examine it may be that these questions are used and we have included a few in this book for this reason.

It is also possible that some questions will be phrased, 'Regarding XYZ, which of the following is true?' This is essentially a true/false question where you know that only one of the options is true, hence if you can answer any four of the options, you can answer the question correctly because even if you only know those that are false you can deduce that the remaining option must be the correct answer.

It is much easier to convert old true/false questions into these formats than proper SBA and as the RCR has a large bank of true/false questions it may be that they choose to do this to make up the number of available questions.

Similarly, there are some topics that lend themselves so well to multiple choice questions that there is always a temptation to examine them because they are easy to test rather than because they are particularly important or useful. We have tried hard to target questions to the important or useful topics and have made efforts to avoid easily constructed but largely irrelevant items, but this too would be a relatively easy way to make up the number of available questions.

No more negative marking: answer every question

You may pass with knowledge alone and the bulk of this book is dedicated to helping you do this. Some candidates, however, – whether through poor preparation, nerves, bad luck or whatever other cause – will find themselves close to passing but stumped by a number of questions and teetering close to but below the pass mark. At this point exam technique really comes into its own and it is a question of 'salvage' – getting whatever you can from the remaining questions and on balance doing better than chance. You don't need to be correct in every guess, just to skew the odds in your favour so you are more likely to be correct than with a blind guess, and with each question you will continue to pull closer to the pass mark and ahead of the pack. Now that negative marking has been scrapped there is no risk of failing through bad luck from poor guessing and everyone should aim to maximise their mark even with the questions they don't understand or of which they are uncertain. Unlike negative marking there is no longer a need to get more right than wrong and it is now quite simple: answer every question.

HOW TO GET A QUESTION RIGHT WHEN YOU DON'T KNOW THE ANSWER

You may be able to narrow the options down through your knowledge of what is being tested alone and pick between them, but even if you know nothing about the topic then you should guess intelligently.

The following methods of exam technique are likely to get you more than the expected 20% on a one from five single best answer question. These questions are difficult to construct properly and you should exploit any weakness in the question for your gain. What an examiner may consider a fault may prove helpful to a candidate with good technique and act as a marker for the right answer, even if you know nothing about the topic being examined. The following tips are presented roughly in descending order of reliability and several may be applicable to a single question.

1   Be suspicious of answers that do not follow from the stem (grammatically or temporally) as they are unlikely to be correct and are probably poor distractors.

2   If there are multiple stems that would have to be correct if one stem was correct, that stem must be wrong; that is, if option A were correct then option B would also have to be correct means that A must be wrong as there can only be one correct answer. (It remains possible that B is the correct answer unless B being correct would also imply that A had to be correct too.) *See* example below.

3   Compare the options and use the vignette for clues to the answer – is there a key difference between them (e.g. histiocytosis and LAM) that you remember which you can work backwards to deduce from the vignette?

4   Look for 'non-homogeneous' (to use medical education jargon) options where one answer is substantially different from the others. This item is probably an incorrect 'filler'. (Beware that it is possible but less likely that it is the correct answer and limited knowledge may help you spot this if the other four options are poor 'fillers'.)

5   You may be able to use one question to work out the answer from another; for example, a vignette may give a clinical history and a radiological finding and then later in the paper a question may ask what finding you would expect in that clinical situation.

6   Look for a cue in the options – longer options with more detail are more likely in a correct answer.

7   Terms that are repeated in question and option make that option more likely to be the correct answer.

8   Normal values or a 'null' option are probably wrong.

9   Convergence: Look for options where some component overlaps; the option with the most overlap with all the other options is more likely correct. This is particularly obvious with a table where the most frequently occurring option in a column is probably correct and by considering all the columns together it may be possible to narrow down the options to a single answer. (Note, however, that when setting the questions in this book we have deliberately drawn up tables where this is not possible, but it is an extra step to use as a possible hint and it may be that some questions creep through without this check happening.)

Option	T Stage	N Stage	M Stage
A	1	2	X
B (More likely)	2	2	0
C	3	2	1
D	1	3	0
E	2	3	0
	T1 or T2 appear twice	N2 appears 3 times	M0 appears 3 times

10   When considering tabulated data think which is the more likely clinical scenario; for example, T2N2M0 is probably more clinically likely than T1N3M0.

11   Beware of absolute terms – medicine has never been an exact science. Such terms – always, invariably, never, etc. – may well be part of a distractor that the examiner has phrased in this way to make it wrong. It is good practice to

think specifically if you know about that option in the condition being tested and whether it is a specific clue as occasionally these terms will be correct, but this is often obvious and is the exception rather than the rule.

12 If you have no idea, there may even be a clue in the order of the answers. When setting the options it is tempting to put the correct option slightly more often first or last and slightly less often at B or D. Clearly, there are easy rigorous ways to overcome this (alphabetical arrangement of the answers, which will be apparent when you look at the paper or use of truly random allocation, which won't).

13 Similarly, the extremes of numerical data are probably more likely to be incorrect.

For an illustration of these features, which have been exaggerated for effect, consider the following question:

> A retired dockworker presents with shortness of breath and is assessed with a chest radiograph. This shows multiple leaf-shaped calcific opacities projected over both lungs. The underlying lungs appear normal. What is the most likely diagnosis?
> a Probably asbestos-related pleural plaques but not asbestosis
> b Asbestosis
> c Mania
> d Disseminated malignancy
> e Metastatic lung cancer

This question has a number of faults. Not only is the correct option (A) obvious but it is longer and more complete than the other options, making it distinctive. The correct option and the incorrect asbestosis are relatively similar compared to the other options, giving a hint that one of them is probably correct. The two options disseminated malignancy and lung cancer are mutually exclusive hence neither can be correct. The final distractor (mania) is entirely non-homogeneous, as the condition bears no relation to the patient's symptom and could not be diagnosed from the investigation in the question.

EXAM TECHNIQUE
Timekeeping

Single best answer questions take some time to read and time is likely to be much tighter than with the true/false format, particularly if you are not very quick at reading written English. Work out how long you have on average per question and at least on the first pass through the paper don't spend much longer than this on any one question. This method will maximise your chances of finishing the paper (and gaining any easy marks towards the end of the question paper) before you return to spend whatever time you have left on the difficult questions. Only spend the extra time on these questions as you go through if you are certain that you will, overall, still have time to complete the paper. Many people like to take a clock and write down the time the exam started and will finish.

We chose 70 questions as the length of the papers in this book to achieve a balance between content and the time required to complete the paper before the Royal College of Radiologists confirmed their plans for the examination. They have very recently announced their intention to include 75 questions in the actual examination and we highlight this so candidates are aware that in the actual exam five more questions will need to be completed in the available time than in the papers in this book.

Order in which to answer questions

There is no obligation to answer the questions in the order in which they are presented and candidates adopt many strategies including missing out those they are unsure of and completing those of which they are certain before returning to the others. Indeed, the vast majority of candidates will miss out at least a few questions on their first pass. When doing this make sure of two things. Firstly, make sure that you make a note somewhere of which question you need to return to. You could have a blank sheet with headings such as 'Need to check' (but reasonably sure), 'It'll come back to me' and 'No idea'. Other people prefer to write on the question paper and circle the question number, draw an arrow in from the margin, or whatever. Similarly, a few will write a similar description for questions where they are so certain that they don't want to go back and waste time checking to remind them to miss out that question if they are checking the paper at the end. Secondly, and most importantly, when you miss out a question make absolutely certain that you put the answer to the next question you answer in the correct place on the answer sheet.

Writing the answers on the question paper or a blank sheet

Some candidates initially note their answers on the question paper or a blank sheet and then transfer them to the answer sheet after they have answered all the questions. This method may appeal to some people particularly if they are apt to change their minds several times and are worried they may 'make a mess' of the exam answer paper, but it is extremely high risk for two reasons. Firstly, errors when under pressure are easy and getting out of sequence with the answers will be catastrophic. Secondly, if you run out of time then rather than having, say, 99% of the paper complete you will have nothing as your answers cannot be handed in until they are transcribed. Hence we would sound a note of caution and advise that if you do choose this method, you should be exceptionally careful to keep the right question with the right answer and to complete the transcription in good time.

If you run out of time

If you run out of time, rapidly fill in any blanks and the remainder of the questions by just guessing the answer. If you really have run out of time it is critically important you mark any answer for every question as quickly as possible, so do not waste time reading the question paper – just guess randomly.

Cardiothoracic and vascular radiology

PAPER 1

1   A 34-year-old female undergoing a contrast swallow is noted to have a smooth anterior indentation on the oesophagram. Which of the following is most likely to be responsible?
a   Right-sided aortic arch
b   Aortic aneurysm
c   Aberrant right subclavian artery
d   Aberrant left pulmonary artery
e   Double aortic arch

2   A 34-year-old female presented with hypertension and an ejection systolic murmur. Which finding is most likely to support a diagnosis of true coarctation compared to pseudocoarctation?
a   Figure '3' sign on angiogram
b   An associated bicuspid aortic valve
c   Rib notching
d   High positioned aortic arch
e   Dilatation of the distal aorta

3   A 72-year-old man presented to his general practitioner with progressive dyspnoea. He has a history of hypertension and is a smoker. The chest radiograph demonstrates mild cardiomegaly and widening of the mediastinum at the level of the aortic arch. After referral to a cardiologist, a contrast-enhanced computed tomography examination was performed which revealed a soft tissue density mass in contact with the aortic arch with a central pool of contrast at the same density as the aorta. The pre-contrast images showed a fine rim of calcification peripherally. What is the most likely diagnosis?
a   Aortic dissection with mediastinal haematoma
b   Bronchogenic carcinoma invading the mediastinum
c   Bronchogenic cyst
d   Lymphadenopathy
e   Atherosclerotic aortic aneurysm

4 A 50-year-old man who is an outpatient had a chest radiograph that demonstrates globular cardiomegaly suspicious of a pericardial effusion. What would be the next appropriate investigation to further investigate this finding?
a Magnetic resonance imaging
b Echocardiogram
c Computed tomography examination
d Electrocardiogram
e Myocardial perfusion scan

5 A 25-year-old female underwent a CT to investigate a history of progressive leg claudication, abdominal pain, night sweats and myalgia. Circumferential thickening of the thoracic and abdominal aortic wall with a stenosis in the thoracic aorta was seen and a magnetic resonance angiogram performed. On short tau inversion recovery (STIR) sequences there is high signal in the aortic wall. What is the most likely diagnosis?
a Behcet's disease
b Acute lymphoblastic leukaemia
c Polyarteritis nodosa
d Takayasu's arteritis
e Giant cell aortitis

6 A previously fit and well 45-year-old male presented with fever, abdominal pain and weight loss. Clinical examination was unremarkable. The erythrocyte sedimentation rate was raised but his leucocyte count was normal. After referral to the surgical team a CT of his abdomen was performed. This showed thickening of the wall of the ascending colon with pericolic fat stranding. Contrast was seen within the superior mesenteric vessel and there was a wedge-shaped area of low attenuation in the spleen. A selective angiogram of the superior mesenteric artery was performed, which demonstrated multiple aneurysms measuring between 1 and 5 mm. What is the most likely diagnosis?
a Ischaemic colitis
b Systemic lupus erythematosus
c Polyarteritis nodosa
d Rheumatoid vasculitis
e Wegener's granulomatosis

7 A 39-year-old male smoker was referred to a cardiologist with chest pain. A cardiac magnetic resonance examination was requested as part of his work-up. This showed patchy multifocal delayed hyperenhancement within the basal interventricular septum. What is the most likely diagnosis?
a Sarcoidosis
b Amyloidosis
c Ischaemic myocardium
d Myocarditis
e Hypertrophic cardiomyopathy

8 A 25-year-old male was referred for a routine testicular screening ultrasound. He is known to have a cardiac myxoma and has multiple pigmented lesions on his face and lips. What is the most likely unifying diagnosis?
a Carney's syndrome
b Peutz-Jeghers syndrome
c Waardenburg's syndrome
d Cronkhite-Canada syndrome
e Gorlin's syndrome

9 Regarding multidetector computed tomography for coronary artery disease, which of the following statements is true?
a It has a low negative predictive value
b It is ideally used in a population with a low pre-test probability of coronary artery disease
c It is accurate in detecting stenosis in small vessels
d The Rockford scoring system is used
e It is less accurate than magnetic resonance imaging in detecting extent of calcification

10 A 58-year-old male who frequently attends the Emergency Department presents with dyspnoea and chest wall pain. His chest radiograph demonstrates cardiomegaly, multiple rib fractures of varying ages and right lower lobe consolidation. What is the most likely unifying diagnosis?
a Chronic alcohol abuse
b Sickle cell anaemia
c Congestive cardiac failure
d Amyloidosis
e X-linked cardioskeletal myopathy

11 A 45-year-old man presents with worsening dyspnoea over a two-year period. Chest radiography demonstrates enlarged central pulmonary arteries and elevation of the cardiac apex. Which of the following is most likely?
a Ventricular septal defect
b Patent ductus arteriosus
c Atrial septal defect
d Partial anomalous pulmonary venous drainage
e Endocardial cushion defect

12 A 56-year-old female was referred to the cardiology outpatient clinic with recent onset exertional dyspnoea. An echocardiogram showed left ventricular dysfunction and a cardiac MRI was requested to identify the cause. Cine images revealed focal hypokinesis in the anteroseptal wall and delayed enhanced images show increased signal in the subendocardium. What is the most likely diagnosis?

a Myocarditis
b Myocardial infarction
c Hypertrophic cardiomyopathy
d Amyloidosis
e Tako-tsubo cardiomyopathy

13 A 56-year-old male patient presented with headache and swelling of his face and neck. A chest radiograph revealed several parenchymal opacities of varying sizes and widening of the superior mediastinum. What is the most likely cause of this presentation?

a Superior vena cava obstruction (SVCO) secondary to metastatic renal cell carcinoma
b SVCO secondary to tuberculous lymphadenopathy
c SVCO secondary to metastatic bronchogenic carcinoma
d SVCO secondary to metastatic thyroid carcinoma
e SVCO secondary to primary pulmonary lymphoma

14 A 59-year-old female patient presented with malaise, chest pain and dyspnoea. Her chest radiograph was normal. An echocardiogram demonstrated a mobile echogenic mass attached to the intra-atrial septum by a stalk. What is the most likely diagnosis?

a Pulmonary embolism
b Papillary fibroelastoma
c Sarcoma
d Fibrovillous adenoma
e Cardiac myxoma

15 A 67-year-old retired musician was admitted to the acute medical ward at 7.00 am with dyspnoea. Examination revealed central cyanosis, tachypnoea and bilateral crepitations, which were most marked at the bases. Initial investigations revealed hypoxia, tachycardia and an abnormal ECG. A chest radiograph demonstrated perihilar alveolar opacification, interstitial thickening, small bi-basal effusions and upper lobe blood diversion. On further questioning it is apparent that the patient had been increasingly breathless for several months and subsequent echocardiography demonstrated cardiomyopathy. What echocardiographic finding would be most suggestive of a restrictive rather than a dilated cause for the cardiomyopathy?

a Decreased systolic function
b Isolated diastolic dysfunction
c Cardiac mural thrombus

d Reduced cardiac output

e Increased LV cavity size

16 You are asked to review a chest radiograph of an 18-year-old female inpatient. The cardiac apex lies on the right side. The aortic knuckle is also seen on the right. Gas within the stomach is seen under the left hemidiaphragm. Otherwise the cardio-mediastinal appearances are unremarkable. The appearance and orientation of the ribs is normal. What is the most likely explanation for these findings?

a Dextrocardia

b Situs invertus

c Situs solitus

d Levoposition due to pectus excavatum

e Asplenia

17 A 43-year-old woman presents with fever, malaise, arthralgia and myalgia. She also complains of pain in her left arm after activity and on examination her left radial pulse is weak. Her ESR is elevated but the other blood tests are unremarkable. A chest radiograph demonstrates an undulating contour of the lateral margin of the descending aorta and CT angiography reveals multifocal areas of thickening and enhancement of the wall of the thoracic aorta and left subclavian artery. Non-occlusive thrombus is seen within the left subclavian artery. What is the most likely diagnosis?

a Polyarteritis nodosa

b Rheumatoid vasculitis

c Churg-Strauss syndrome

d Microscopic polyangiitis

e Takayasu's disease

18 A 27-year-old female with gradually worsening exercise tolerance had a chest radiograph as part of her work-up. She has a past history of rheumatic heart disease. The chest radiograph shows an increased cardiothoracic diameter with a double right heart border and upper lobe blood diversion. There was an area of calcification projected over the cardiac shadow. Which valvular condition is most likely?

a Aortic stenosis

b Aortic regurgitation

c Mitral stenosis

d Tricuspid stenosis

e Tricuspid regurgitation

19 A 32-year-old man with known hereditary haemorrhagic telangiectasia (Osler-Weber-Rendu syndrome) was admitted for elective embolisation of a pulmonary arteriovenous malformation. What would be the most appropriate material with which to embolise this lesion?
    a Coils
    b PVA particles
    c Glue
    d Lipidol
    e Alcohol

20 A 63-year-old gentleman was diagnosed with a q-wave acute myocardial infarction and underwent a cardiac MRI the following day. What is the most likely signal intensity of the infarcted region on T2-weighted imaging?
    a Signal void
    b Low
    c Isointense
    d High
    e Variable

21 A 62-year-old gentleman with exertional dyspnoea was referred by his cardiologist for a stress cardiac MR study. His medical history includes hyperlipidaemia, asthma and hypertension. Which of the following pharmacological stress agents is best suited for this patient?
    a Adenosine
    b Dobutamine
    c Atenolol
    d Verapamil
    e Dopamine

22 A 62-year-old gentleman presented with syncopal episodes and intermittent pain and paraesthesia in his right hand especially when exerting his right arm. An MRI demonstrated obstruction of his right subclavian artery. Where in the artery is the obstruction most likely to be located?
    a First part of the artery, at its origin
    b First part of the artery, just distal to the right vertebral artery
    c Second part of the artery, just distal to the deep cervical artery
    d Second part of the artery, just proximal to dorsal scapular artery
    e Just lateral to the lateral border of the scalenus anterior muscle

23 A 39-year-old gentleman with frequent respiratory tract infections and recent onset stridor was assessed with a CT of his thorax. A vessel was seen passing above the right main stem bronchus and coursing between the trachea and oesophagus. The trachea was deviated to the left and there was atelectasis in the right upper lobe. Which abnormal vessel is most likely to be present?
    a Aberrant left pulmonary artery
    b Aberrant right pulmonary artery

c Double aortic arch
d Aberrant right subclavian artery
e Aberrant left subclavian artery

24 A 55-year-old hypertensive diabetic presented with chest pain and was found to have a myocardial infarct of his interventricular septum and apex. In which vessel territory is this area most likely to lie?
a Left anterior descending artery
b Left circumflex artery
c Posterior descending artery
d Conus artery
e Acute marginal branches of the right coronary artery

25 At one week a neonate developed lower-extremity cyanosis. Their chest radiograph showed an enlarged heart with increased pulmonary vasculature. The aorta had a figure '3' appearance. What is the most common associated abnormality?
a Bicuspid aortic valve
b Ventricular septal defect
c Atrial septal defect
d Cerebral berry aneurysms
e Mycotic aneurysms in the descending aorta

26 A patient is awaiting investigation and treatment of a superficial neck mass, suspicious for non-Hodgkin's lymphoma. Their chest radiograph shows bilateral hilar lymphadenopathy. When is the best time to perform PET CT in view of gaining a histological diagnosis and commencing treatment?
a Wait 1 week after neck dissection
b Wait 4 weeks after neck dissection
c Wait 4–6/52 after start of chemotherapy
d Within 1 week of commencing chemotherapy
e Wait 4–6 weeks after starting radiotherapy

27 A 40-year-old female presented with shortness of breath and her chest radio-graph was normal. She underwent a ventilation/perfusion study to investigate a possible pulmonary embolus. This showed two small, unmatched subseg-mental defects in the left apical region. The ventilation images are normal. What is the correct report for this study?
a Normal study
b Very low probability
c Low probability
d High probability
e Intermediate probability

28 A patient with a lung cancer measuring 3.5 cm in their right upper lobe 4 cm from the mediastinal structures with 1-cm nodes in the right hilum and a 3-mm nodule in the right lower lobe underwent PET CT for further staging following a standard CT. The primary tumour is avid and further uptake of over 2.5 SUV is seen in the nodes of ipsilateral hilum. Further uptake is seen bilaterally in the supraclavicular region in a linear distribution although no associated soft tissue mass is seen on the corresponding diagnostic CT. The small nodule in the right lower lobe is not well visualised on PET and no uptake is seen related to it. What is the most likely TNM staging based on the PET scan?
a T1N2M0
b T2N1Mx
c T2N1M1
d T1N2Mx
e T1N1M0

29 An infant who is failing to thrive with difficulty feeding presents with increased work of breathing. A chest radiograph shows moderate cardiomegaly, bulky pulmonary vessels and fluid in the fissures. What is the most likely diagnosis?
a Atrial septal defect
b Ventricular septal defect
c Patent ductus arteriosus
d Pulmonary artery stenosis
e Aortic coarctation

30 A routine baby check on a neonate born at term reveals bounding peripheral pulses and a continuous murmur, loudest under the clavicle. What is the most likely diagnosis?
a Patent ductus arteriosus
b Ventricular septal defect
c Atrio-ventricular septal defect
d Pulmonary stenosis
e Transposition of the great arteries

31 A 32-year-old man developed a low-grade fever and weight loss. He was previously well and had never smoked. CT shows lymphadenopathy on both sides of the diaphragm and a sample taken at mediastinoscopy showed Reed-Sternberg cells. There were no further positive findings in the rest of the thorax or abdomen. Where in the thorax is the lymphadenopathy most likely?
a Anterior mediastinum
b Middle mediastinum
c Posterior mediastinum
d Superior mediastinum
e Hilar nodes

32 A 64-year-old non-smoker presents to his GP with progressive dyspnoea. His chest radiograph demonstrates a peripheral lung mass. What is the most likely histological type of carcinoma?

    a Squamous cell carcinoma

    b Small cell lung carcinoma

    c Bronchoalveolar cell carcinoma

    d Large cell carcinoma

    e Adenocarcinoma

33 A patient with a known malignancy presented with acute shortness of breath. The attending physician requested CT pulmonary angiogram to exclude a pulmonary embolus. A filling defect was seen in the left lower pulmonary artery with a wedge-shaped collapse distal to it. Which primary tumour is most frequently associated with pulmonary embolism?

    a Lung carcinoma

    b Hepatocellular carcinoma

    c Gastric carcinoma

    d Ovarian cystadenoma

    e Prostate carcinoma

34 A 75-year-old gentleman who had worked in the construction industry had a chest radiograph prior to an elective cholecystectomy. Multiple calcified pleural plaques were visible bilaterally with lower zone predominant reticular opacification. What is the most likely pleural manifestation of this disease?

    a Diffuse pleural thickening

    b Pleural effusion

    c Focal pleural plaques

    d Pleural calcification

    e Mesothelioma

35 A patient with long-standing severe rheumatoid arthritis developed progressive dyspnoea. What is the most frequent intra-thoracic manifestation of the disease?

    a Pleural disease

    b Interstitial fibrosis

    c Bronchiectasis

    d Bronchiolitis obliterans

    e Pulmonary nodules

36 A 38-year-old female of West African decent presented with a fever, malaise and large joint arthralgia. She was also noted to have erythema nodosum. Her calcium levels were elevated and her chest radiograph showed bilateral nodular pulmonary hila. What is the most likely diagnosis?
   a Familial Mediterranean fever
   b Malaria
   c Acute sarcoidosis
   d Severe acute respiratory syndrome (SARS)
   e Lymphomatoid granulomatosis

37 The chest radiograph of a severely dyspnoeic patient with AIDS showed bilateral diffuse interstitial and airspace infiltrates with a symmetrical peri-hilar distribution. What would you expect the CD4 count to be (in cells/microlitre)?
   a 1000
   b 750
   c 600
   d 400
   e 150

38 A chest radiograph taken of an adult female with underlying chronic lung disease demonstrates hyperinflated lungs, patchy upper lobe consolidation and several 1- to 2-cm ring shadows in a predominantly upper lobe distribution. A recent full blood count showed an eosinophilia. What is the most likely diagnosis?
   a Hypersensitivity pneumonia
   b Eosinophilic pneumonia
   c Allergic bronchopulmonary aspergillosis
   d Tuberculosis
   e Lipoid pneumonia

39 A 20-year-old male presented to the Emergency Department with chest pain. A chest radiograph demonstrated an abnormal density behind the heart and while his symptoms resolved rapidly the abnormality persisted on repeat imaging. A CT showed it to be a mass within the left lower lobe with a systemic arterial supply. What additional finding would make a diagnosis of intralobar bronchopulmonary sequestration more likely than an extralobar type?
   a The presence of multiple small systemic feeding arteries
   b An associated diaphragmatic hernia
   c A more solid appearance to the mass
   d Separate pleural layer around the mass
   e Drainage via pulmonary veins

40 A previously healthy adult male has been diagnosed with active pulmonary tuberculosis infection. What feature on imaging would suggest primary rather than reactivated pulmonary tuberculosis?
a Cavity formation
b Calcification
c Tuberculoma formation
d Non-specific pneumonitis
e Fibrosis and distortion of lung architecture

41 A 56-year-old man presented with recurrent episodes of fever, dry cough and dyspnoea. On specific questioning he states he breeds pigeons. What feature would make the diagnosis of extrinsic allergic alveolitis (EAA) less likely?
a Pleural effusion
b A normal chest radiograph
c Fibrosis of middle and lower zones
d Traction bronchiectasis
e Diffuse ground-glass attenuation on high resolution CT

42 A 45-year-old female presented with progressive dyspnoea. A chest radiograph demonstrated reticular densities with preserved lung volumes. An HRCT showed uniform cysts throughout the lung with normal intervening lung. What is the most likely diagnosis?
a Tuberous sclerosis
b Lymphangiomyomatosis
c Histiocytosis
d Tuberculosis
e Cystic fibrosis

43 A 50-year-old man was admitted feeling unwell and multiple ill-defined nodules of varying sizes within both lungs were visible on his chest radiograph. These were suspected to be lung metastases. What is the most likely primary tumour?
a Testicular teratoma
b Renal cell carcinoma
c Thyroid carcinoma
d Melanoma
e Pancreatic carcinoma

44 A 30-year-old male presented with night sweats and weight loss. A chest radiograph revealed widening of the right paratracheal space and a CT demonstrated extensive lymphadenopathy within the thorax but no sub-diaphragmatic involvement. In view of a likely diagnosis of lymphoma, what would make non-Hodgkin's lymphoma more likely than Hodgkin's lymphoma?

   a Abnormal T-cells on lymph node biopsy
   b Incidence
   c Pleural effusion
   d Normal chest radiograph six months previously
   e Involvement of principally the hilar and subcarinal lymph nodes

45 A patient who was known to have HIV presented with shortness of breath and underwent further investigations. Their CD4 count was 208 cells per cu mm. What AIDS-defining illness would be most likely with this CD4 count?

   a Lymphoma
   b Histoplasmosis
   c Kaposi's sarcoma
   d *Pneumocystis carinii* pneumonia
   e Pulmonary CMV

46 A 54-year-old female presented with progressive dyspnoea and diffuse pulmonary opacities on her chest radiograph. An HRCT revealed inter-lobular septal thickening bibasally. What further findings would suggest a diagnosis of lymphangitis carcinomatosis rather than cardiogenic pulmonary oedema?

   a Nodular interlobular septal thickening
   b Pleural fluid
   c Ground-glass opacification
   d Centrilobular nodules
   e Mediastinal lymphadenopathy

47 A 50-year-old man who presented with progressive dyspnoea had a chest radiograph that demonstrated multiple opacities between 0.5 and 2 mm in size, which were noted to be more dense than soft tissue. Which of the following diagnoses is most likely?

   a Fungal infection such as histoplasmosis
   b Coal miners' pneumoconiosis
   c Sarcoidosis
   d Acute extrinsic allergic alveolitis
   e Silicosis

48 A 32-year-old male was found by the roadside in respiratory distress. There is very little clinical history, but his condition deteriorated in the Emergency Department and he was intubated, ventilated and transferred to ICU.

His initial chest radiograph showed widespread alveolar infiltrates of a non-specific nature. He had a CT of the chest with high-resolution sections. What additional finding would be most compatible with a diagnosis of adult respiratory distress syndrome?

a The presence of pneumatoceles

b Predominantly dependent abnormality

c Ground glass attenuation

d Pneumothorax

e Septal nodularity

49 A 64-year-old female was seen in the Emergency Department for dyspnoea. She was otherwise fit and well and had no significant past medical history. A full blood count showed a mild neutrophilia and a chest radiograph revealed significant elevation of the right hemidiaphragm. What is the most likely cause?

a Herpes zoster infection

b Previous iatrogenic trauma

c Compression of the phrenic nerve by a tumour

d Peripheral neuropathy secondary to cervical spondylosis

e Compression of the phrenic nerve caused by a thoracic aortic aneurysm

50 A 40-year-old schoolteacher presented with a non-productive cough, dyspnoea and low-grade pyrexia. She has never smoked. The CXR demonstrated several bilateral areas of patchy consolidation which were confirmed on HRCT and shown to be in a mainly sub-pleural distribution. In addition there is also patchy ground-glass change and small (<5 mm) centrilobular nodules). What is the most likely diagnosis?

a Bronchoalveolar cell carcinoma

b Histoplasmosis

c Sarcoidosis

d Cryptogenic organising pneumonia

e Multifocal streptococcal pneumonia

51 At the weekly respiratory multidisciplinary team meeting you are asked to review a chest radiograph and CT of a 39-year-old man who presented with cough, fever, dyspnoea and chest pain. Blood biochemistry had demonstrated renal impairment. The imaging reveals bilateral reticulonodular interstitial opacification. The nodules vary in size, and the larger nodules show cavitation. What is the most likely diagnosis?

a Wegener's granulomatosis

b Eosinophilic pneumonia

c Systemic lupus erythematosus (SLE)

d Multiple pulmonary emboli

e Goodpasture's syndrome

52 A 32-year-old artist presented with chest pain and dyspnoea. Physical examination was unremarkable but blood gas analysis showed her to be markedly hypoxic and a pulmonary embolus was suspected. A CT pulmonary angiogram (CTPA) was performed with bolus tracking (threshold triggering); however, the pulmonary arterial contrast opacification was sub-optimal. The intravenous cannula is well sited and there is no overt sign of swelling around the cannula site. The patient took a deep breath just prior to the scan and the scan appeared to trigger appropriately with the region of interest (ROI) sited over the main pulmonary artery. What is the most likely cause for the sub-optimal opacification of the pulmonary vessels?
   a Left to right shunt
   b Contrast extravasation at the injection site
   c Right to left shunt
   d Dilution of opacified blood with unopacified blood
   e Hypodynamic circulation

53 You have been asked to review a chest radiograph by a junior doctor. The image demonstrates subtle hazy opacification of the upper part of the lower zone of the right lung. The right atrial border is indistinct and the horizontal fissure runs from the right hilum to the eighth rib in the mid axillary line. What is the most plausible explanation for these findings?
   a Middle lobe collapse
   b Middle lobe consolidation
   c Pectus excavatum
   d Right lower lobe mediobasal segment consolidation
   e Right lower lobe anteriobasal segment consolidation

54 A 62-year-old widow presented to the Neurology Clinic with fatigue and weakness, particularly after minimal exertion. Cranial nerve examination revealed rapid fatigability of the facial muscles and her chest radiograph showed mediastinal widening. The patient then underwent contrast enhanced CT of the chest. Which of the following findings best fits the given clinical scenario?
   a Diffuse mediastinal adenopathy and a widespread interstitial thickening
   b Retrosternal goitre demonstrating areas of necrosis and haemorrhage with avid contrast enhancement
   c Isolated homogeneous soft tissue mass within the anterior mediastinum outlined by fat
   d Diffuse, invasive mass containing areas of haemorrhage and calcification encasing the major vessels
   e Large, eccentric aortic arch aneurysm

55 A 46-year-old patient presented with a long history of dyspnoea, cough and fatigue. A chest radiograph demonstrated established fibrotic changes. What feature most suggests a diagnosis of idiopathic pulmonary fibrosis/usual interstitial pneumonia (UIP) rather than non-specific interstitial pneumonia (NSIP)?

a Traction bronchiectasis
b Septal thickening
c Ground-glass opacification
d Honeycombing
e Reduced lung volumes

56 A 46-year-old woman presented to the Respiratory Clinic with a two-year history of cough, dyspnoea, fatigue and weight loss. She was under concurrent investigation by the rheumatologists for Sjögren's disease. Examination was unremarkable apart from bilateral inspiratory crepitations. A chest radiograph revealed a reticular pattern of opacification and subsequent HRCT showed septal thickening, bilateral diffuse ground-glass shadowing and poorly defined centrilobular nodules. What is the most likely potential pathological finding on lung biopsy?

a Haemorrhagic alveolar infiltrate
b *Aspergillus* spores
c Neutrophilic alveolar infiltrate
d Lymphoid interstitial infiltrate
e Histeocytic alveolar infiltrate

57 A retired railway worker underwent plain chest radiography and CT scanning. What appearance would be most in keeping with benign asbestos-related pleural plaque disease?

a Asymmetric pleural thickening of the right lung, predominantly involving the mediastinal pleural surface. No calcification is evident; however, there is a moderately large pleural effusion.
b Bilateral focal pleural thickening involving the apices and costophrenic angles, but sparing the diaphragms. Most of the plaques are calcified.
c Bilateral focal pleural thickening predominantly affecting the diaphragms and lower thorax, sparing the apices, costophrenic angles and mediastinal pleura. Only a few of the plaques are calcified.
d Bilateral focal pleural thickening involving the lower thorax and sparing the costophrenic angles, diaphragms, mediastinal pleura and apices. Most of the plaques are calcified.
e Bilateral focal pleural thickening involving the costophrenic angles and lower thorax, but sparing the diaphragms, mediastinal pleura and apices. Only a few of the plaques are calcified.

58 A 40-year-old man presented to the Respiratory Clinic with a gradual onset of dyspnoea, weight loss, cough and haemoptysis. He was tachypnoeic at rest with crepitations on auscultation. His full blood count and renal profile were normal. A chest radiograph showed bilateral, patchy hazy opacification and there was a 'crazy paving' pattern of attenuation on HRCT with additional sparse patches of consolidation. There was no adenopathy, cardiomegaly or effusion and lung biopsy was performed. The interstitium was normal but there was filling of the alveoli with lipid and proteinacious material. What is the most likely diagnosis?

  a Sarcoidosis
  b Left heart failure and pulmonary oedema
  c Goodpasture's syndrome
  d Wegener's granulomatosis
  e Alveolar proteinosis

59 A 60-year-old man has chronic obstructive pulmonary disease (COPD). He has a long smoking history and is being considered for lung volume reduction surgery (LVRS). What pattern of disease would give the best chance of a successful outcome following LRVS?

  a Mild, predominantly upper and mid zone paraseptal emphysema
  b Severe lower zone bullous emphysema and mild upper zone paraseptal emphysema
  c Severe upper zone bullous emphysema with relatively spared lower zones
  d Severe upper zone bullous emphysema with moderate lower zone centrilobular emphysema
  e Severe centrilobular emphysema affecting all zones

60 You are asked to perform a chest ultrasound and diagnostic aspiration on a 50-year-old patient with a history of recent pneumonia. The attending physician is concerned as the patient has developed a pleural effusion and remains febrile and unwell despite four days of intravenous antibiotics. What findings are most in keeping with a parapneumonic empyema?

  a Simple pleural effusion and underlying atelectasis on ultrasound. Biochemical/cytological analysis: ph 7.4, lymphocytes ++
  b Septated effusion and underlying consolidation on ultrasound. Biochemical/cytological analysis: ph 7.2, lymphocytes +
  c Simple effusion with underlying consolidation on ultrasound. Biochemical/cytological analysis: ph 7.7, neutrophils ++
  d Septated effusion with underlying atelectasis on ultrasound. Biochemical/cytological analysis: ph 7.4, neutrophils ++, lymphocytes +
  e Septated effusion with underlying consolidation on ultrasound. Biochemical/cytological analysis: ph 7.1, neutrophils ++

61 A 42-year-old man became dyspnoeic two days after a road traffic accident where, among other injuries, he sustained a pelvic, left femoral and right humeral fracture. On examination he was febrile, cyanosed and confused. A number of petechial haemorrhages on his chest and abdomen were noted and you are contacted to review his chest radiograph as it appears normal. What is the most likely diagnosis?

a Pulmonary embolism
b Fat embolism
c Disseminated intravascular coagulation
d Bacterial septicaemia
e Adult respiratory distress syndrome

62 A 62-year-old female patient became unwell 10 days following right lung transplantation. She was short of breath, febrile and lethargic and her oxygen saturations had deteriorated over the previous three days. Her chest radiograph showed heterogeneous peri-hilar airspace opacification, septal thickening and a right pleural effusion. The heart size was unchanged compared to previous radiographs and the upper lobe pulmonary vessels were not distended. Transbronchial lung biopsy showed a mononuclear cell infiltrate and alveolar oedema. What is the most likely cause for the patient's dyspnoea?

a Biventricular heart failure
b Post-transplantation staphylococcal infection
c Bronchiolitis obliterans syndrome
d Reperfusion oedema
e Acute transplant rejection

63 An 82-year-old man with worsening symptoms of lower limb arterial insufficiency underwent MR angiography which demonstrated a short superficial femoral artery stenosis. On transfer to the intervention suite an 18-gauge intravenous cannula was sited in his antecubital fossa and he was given 2 L per minute oxygen via nasal cannulae. A femoral catheter was inserted and shortly after the first diagnostic images he complained of feeling unwell and developed facial swelling and an audible wheeze. What should be your first action?

a Call for the resuscitation team
b Give intravenous adrenaline
c Give intravenous hydrocortisone
d Remove the femoral arterial catheter
e Site a large-bore intravenous cannula

64 A 70-kg patient with no relevant comorbidities underwent an abdominal percutaneous drain insertion. At the start of the procedure 10 mL of 1% lidocaine hydrochloride was infiltrated subcutaneously. The patient developed further pain as dilators and a stiff guidewire were inserted. How much more 1% lidocaine can safely be administered?

   a None
   b 5 mL
   c 10 mL
   d 20 mL
   e 40 mL

65 A 21-year-old man who received a live-related renal transplant became oliguric on the third post-operative day. An ultrasound was arranged and the renal artery resistive index was measured at 0.7. What is the most appropriate interpretation of this result?

   a Normal transplant
   b Acute tubular necrosis
   c Acute rejection
   d Calcineurin inhibitor nephrotoxicity
   e Polyomavirus (BK) infection

66 When planning an endovascular stenting procedure, the internal luminal diameter of the common femoral artery is measured at 6 mm. Assuming that this measurement is accurate and that the vessel will not stretch, what is the largest size vascular catheter that could theoretically be introduced into this vessel?

   a 2 Fr
   b 6 Fr
   c 12 Fr
   d 18 Fr
   e 24 Fr

67 An elderly former smoker with worsening ischaemic symptoms in both legs underwent diagnostic lower limb angiography. Independent of the signs and symptoms of his disease, what is the most likely site of atherosclerotic disease in the lower limb?

   a Iliac artery
   b Common femoral artery
   c Superficial femoral artery
   d Popliteal artery
   e Tibial artery

68 A 31-year-old man developed fever and haematuria. Physical examination revealed multiple subcutaneous nodules and blood tests that his ESR was raised. Following an abnormal renal ultrasound and CT he underwent renal angiography. Multiple small intrarenal aneurysms were demonstrated. What is the most likely diagnosis?

a Atherosclerosis

b Ehlers-Danlos syndrome

c Fibromuscular dysplasia

d Polyarteritis nodosa

e Von Hippel-Lindau disease

69 A 17-year-old student presented with an acutely ischaemic left calf and foot and on further questioning he described several months of claudication in his left calf which was worse during periods of prolonged standing. He also reluctantly admitted to a single episode of intravenous drug use through the antecubital fossa. Lower limb arteriography demonstrated stenosis and post-stenotic dilatation of the popliteal artery, which was noted to be deviated medially within the popliteal fossa. What is the most likely diagnosis?

a Atherosclerosis

b Baker's cyst

c Buerger's disease

d Mycotic aneurysm

e Popliteal entrapment

70 A patient underwent endovascular repair of an abdominal aortic aneurysm. After the endograft had been successfully sited a check angiogram showed opacification of the aneurysm sac by retrograde flow through the inferior mesenteric artery. What type of endoleak is this?

a Type I endoleak

b Type II endoleak

c Type III endoleak

d Type IV endoleak

e Type V endoleak (endotension)

Cardiothoracic and vascular radiology

PAPER 2

1   A 46-year-old male who was in a high-speed road traffic accident presents acutely to the Emergency Department. He has severe chest pain radiating to his back and is haemodynamically unstable. What finding on an anterior posterior chest radiograph is most specific for acute thoracic aortic injury?
    a Widening of the mediastinum
    b Widened right paratracheal stripe
    c Indistinct aortic arch contour
    d Obscuration of the aortopulmonary window
    e Right-sided haemothorax

2   You are asked to review a chest radiograph following a pacemaker insertion. The leads have been placed via the left subclavian approach and pass down the left mediastinal border before forming a loop with the tip projected over the right ventricle. What is the most likely explanation?
    a Partial anomalous pulmonary venous return
    b An atrial septal defect
    c A persistent left superior vena cava
    d A ventricular septal defect
    e Normal appearance, no abnormality

3   A three-week-old baby had a chest radiograph to investigate tachypnoea and mild cyanosis which showed cardiomegaly. An echocardiogram revealed a dilated right atrium and abnormal tricuspid valve with a small, dysplastic but functioning right ventricle. What is the most likely diagnosis?
    a Tricuspid atresia
    b Ebstein's anomaly
    c Myocarditis
    d An atrial septal defect
    e Cor triatriatum

4   A 75-year-old female with dyspnoea had a chest radiograph on admission to the acute medical ward. This showed cardiomegaly with a prominent atrial appendage, a double heart border, a fine ring of calcification behind the cardiac shadow and prominent upper lobe blood vessels. What is the most likely diagnosis?

a A ventricular septal defect
b Mitral valve stenosis
c Ischaemic heart disease
d Aortic root dilatation
e Left ventricular aneurysm

5   A patient with extensive, multi-system arterial disease was scheduled for a lower limb vascular study and intervention. Due to their comorbidities carbon dioxide was considered as a contrast agent rather than iodinated contrast. When should carbon dioxide not be used?

a Intra-arterially below the diaphragm
b Intra-arterially in suspected arteritis
c Intravenously in the presence of an inferior vena cava filter
d Intravenously in Eisenmenger's syndrome
e Intravenously in the presence of a deep venous thrombosis

6   A 64-year-old male smoker was seen by the vascular surgical team in the outpatient clinic with increasing unilateral lower limb claudication. A duplex ultrasound showed a stenosis within the left popliteal artery. What is the most likely cause?

a Popliteal artery entrapment syndrome
b Post-traumatic stenosis
c Cystic adventitial disease
d Atherosclerosis
e Emboli

7   A 44-year-old female presented to the Emergency Department in heart failure. An electrocardiogram demonstrated Q waves in lead III and a VF consistent with a previous inferior myocardial infarction. A coronary angiogram was then performed. Which vessel is most likely to be responsible for the infarct?

a Left main stem
b Left anterior descending artery
c Obtuse marginal artery
d Right coronary artery
e Circumflex artery

8 A 34-year-old male presented to the Cardiology team with syncopal episodes and a family history of premature sudden death. A cardiac magnetic resonance examination was requested which showed a dilated right ventricle with a reduced ejection fraction but a normal left ventricle. There was also high signal within the right ventricular free wall on T1-weighted imaging, suggesting fatty replacement. What is the most likely diagnosis?

    a Uhl's syndrome
    b Brugada syndrome
    c Arrhythmogenic right ventricular dysplasia
    d Hypertrophic cardiomyopathy
    e Right ventricular outflow tract tachycardia

9 A 43-year-old male presented to the Cardiology team with a long history of coronary heart disease. His chest radiograph demonstrated enlargement of the left ventricular apex. What characteristic would make a diagnosis of a true ventricular aneurysm more likely than a false aneurysm?

    a A mouth considerably smaller than the maximal diameter
    b No myocardial fibres in the wall
    c An aneurysm that protruded only in systole
    d A previous history of myocardial infarction
    e Thrombus within the aneurysm

10 A 57-year-old man with diabetes mellitus presented with anterior chest pain on minimal exertion and an exercise tolerance test was positive. Cardiac angiography demonstrated 70% stenosis of the circumflex, 90% stenosis of the left anterior descending and complete occlusion of the right coronary arteries. It was agreed with the patient that coronary artery bypass surgery was appropriate. Which of the following native grafts is most appropriate for bypassing the left anterior descending artery?

    a Saphenous vein
    b Left internal mammary artery
    c Left superior epigastric artery
    d Radial vein
    e An intercostal artery

11 A 57-year-old woman presented with reduced exercise tolerance and shortness of breath. No specific abnormality was found on clinical examination. Chest radiography showed enlarged central pulmonary arteries and subsequent chest CT confirmed pulmonary artery enlargement and also showed right ventricular dilation. What additional feature would make chronic thromboembolism a more likely diagnosis than systemic to pulmonary circulation shunting?

    a Pleural effusion
    b Interstitial septal lines
    c Mosaic attenuation

d Flattening of the interventricular septum

e Reflux of contrast into the inferior vena cava

12 A 55-year-old female presented to the Emergency Department with acute central chest pain and shortness of breath. Her daughter had died recently following a post-partum haemorrhage. She was hypotensive with signs of left cardiac failure and her troponin T was elevated. Coronary angiography demonstrated normal coronary arteries and cardiac MRI was performed. This revealed apical hypokinesis and dilatation with normal basal function. There was no myocardial delayed hyperenhancement. Subsequent echocardiography 12 weeks later showed improved left ventricular function. What is the most likely diagnosis?

a Myocardial infarction involving the left anterior descending artery

b Myocarditis

c Hypertrophic cardiomyopathy

d Coronary artery spasm

e Tako-tsubo cardiomyopathy

13 A 65-year-old man with tearing chest pain radiating to his back was investigated with a contrast enhanced CT of his thorax which demonstrated an intimal flap separating the aortic lumen into two separate channels. The flap was seen to originate just distal to the origin of the left subclavian artery and to extend into the left common iliac artery. An aortic dissection is diagnosed. What is the appropriate Stanford classification?

a Stanford type 1

b Stanford type 2

c Stanford type 3

d Stanford type A

e Stanford type B

14 A 47-year-old lady presented with sudden onset right hemiparesis after lifting a heavy shopping bag. CT of her brain demonstrated two foci of low attenuation within the posterior frontal lobe and anterior frontal lobe adjacent to the interhemispheric fissure on the left which involved both white and grey matter. In addition she was also noted to have an erythematous, swollen left calf which was confirmed with a Doppler study to be due to thrombus within the superficial femoral vein. What is the next most appropriate radiological investigation?

a CT venography

b CT arterography

c Echocardiography

d Abdominal ultrasound

e MRI brain

15 A patient undergoing echocardiography for an acyanotic shunt had the following findings on imaging: dilated left atrium and ventricle, dilated right ventricle, undilated right atrium and undilated aorta. What is the most likely cause of the shunt?

   a Ostium primum atrial septal defect (ASD)
   b Ventricular septal defect (VSD)
   c Patent foramen ovale
   d Ostium secundum ASD
   e Patent ductus arteriosus (PDA)

16 A 57-year-old solicitor presented with a swollen left calf. She is on hormone replacement therapy and has a history of pulmonary embolism. What ultrasound feature is most in keeping with a diagnosis of deep vein thrombosis?

   a Venous distension on Valsalva
   b Increased flow within the superficial femoral artery on squeezing the calf
   c Decreased flow in superficial veins and deep collaterals
   d Phasic flow with respiration
   e Loss of phasic flow on Valsalva

17 A 23-year-old intravenous drug abuser presented to the Emergency Department with fever and swelling in his left groin. He was also noted to be short of breath at rest with peripheral cyanosis. A chest radiograph demonstrated widespread bilateral foci of consolidation. Ultrasound of his left groin demonstrated a superficial abscess with non-occlusive thrombus in the left common femoral vein. An echocardiogram performed by a cardiologist showed an echogenic intracardiac mass. What is the best explanation for these findings?

   a Tricuspid valve endocarditis and septic pulmonary emboli
   b Intracardiac bland thrombus and *Mycoplasma* pneumonia
   c Intracardiac bland thrombus and bland pulmonary emboli
   d Pulmonary valve endocarditis and septic pulmonary emboli
   e Mitral valve endocarditis and *Mycoplasma* pneumonia

18 A 25-year-old presented with shortness of breath after minimal exercise. His general practitioner (GP) examined his cardiovascular system and noted a harsh ejection systolic murmur in the left parasternal region. No other murmurs were detected and there were no other positive clinical findings. His chest radiograph showed calcification in the region of the aortic valve. Which of the following is the most likely aetiology?

   a Congenital bicuspid aortic valve
   b Aortic valve atherosclerosis
   c Rheumatic valve disease
   d Previous endocarditis
   e Patent ductus arteriosus

19 A 45-year-old gentleman underwent a contrast-enhanced CT scan of the thorax. His main pulmonary artery has a diameter greater than ascending aorta and the central pulmonary arteries are calcified. The peripheral pulmonary arteries have a pruned appearance. What is the likely pulmonary artery pressure?

a 0 mmHg
b 5 mmHg
c 10 mmHg
d 15 mmHg
e 25 mmHg

20 A 73-year-old man underwent a contrast-enhanced cardiac MR examination. His ECG had not changed over the last six months and showed Q waves in leads II, III and aVF. When would you expect peak differential enhancement of the myocardium in the right coronary artery territory following administration of iodinated contrast?

a No enhancement will occur
b Within 10 seconds
c 20–30 seconds
d 60–90 seconds
e 10–15 minutes

21 A 42-year-old female presented with recurrent chest infections and exertional dyspnoea. She had recently also developed atrial fibrillation and suffered an ischaemic neurological event. Her chest radiograph showed a large heart with a small-looking aorta and echocardiography showed paradoxical movement of the interventricular septum. What is the most likely cardiac abnormality?

a Coarctation of the aorta
b Patent ductus arteriosus
c Ostium secundum atrial septal defect
d Rheumatic mitral stenosis
e Pulmonary stenosis

22 A 65-year-old gentleman presented with syncopal episodes and intermittent pain and paraesthesia in his left hand when he exerted his left upper limb. A Doppler ultrasound demonstrated a stenosis of the left subclavian artery. In which artery would flow reversal be most likely?

a Right common carotid artery
b Right vertebral artery
c Right axillary artery
d Left vertebral artery
e Left subclavian artery

23 A 52-year-old female underwent a follow-up contrast-enhanced CT of her thorax after an episode of viral pericarditis. There was a well-demarcated rounded mass in the paracardiac region. The attenuation was 38 HU (hypodense to myocardium). Where is this mass most likely to be situated?

a Right costophrenic angle
b Anterior to the right ventricle
c Right cardiophrenic angle
d Left cardiophrenic angle
e Posterior mediastinum

24 An individual underwent a stent graft repair of an infra-renal aneurysm a day prior. He presents for a follow-up CT aortogram. A blush of contrast is seen near the end of the stent graft. Which type of endoleak is most compatible with the CT aortogram finding?

a Type I
b Type II
c Type III
d Type IV
e This is a normal finding within 24–48 hours after stent grafting

25 With regard to imaging with PET-CT and the use of F-18 labelled FDG, which of the following is the most accurate statement relating to the behaviour of the radioisotope and acquisition of counts?

a F-18 has a half-life of approximately 60 minutes
b F-18 decays by electron capture
c Annihilation with an electron produces photons with an energy of 115 mBq
d The point source resolution of PET is approx 1 mm
e The dominant annihilation photon interaction in tissue is Compton scatter

26 A patient had a cardiac stress Myoview study and the nurse supervising the study was concerned that he could not continue. What would indicate that terminating the study is the appropriate thing to do?

a Mild chest discomfort
b Mild dizziness
c ST segment depression of 1 mm
d Increase in systolic blood pressure from baseline by 40 mmHg
e Increase in diastolic blood pressure above 120 mmHg

27 A 59-year-old lady with no previous cardiac history presented with intermittent chest pain on exertion not typical of cardiac pain. Her chest radiograph was normal and she is not taking any cardiac medication. She is otherwise well except for bilateral osteoarthritis in the knees. What is the best form of imaging to assess for cardiac ischaemia?

a Tc Myoview rest and chemical stress
b Tc Myoview rest only
c Electrocardiogram
d Exercise tolerance test with electrocardiogram
e Cardiac gated CT

28 A 29-week pregnant patient presented with shortness of breath and hypoxia with pleuritic chest pain. Her chest radiograph was normal and no concurrent cardiopulmonary disease was present. Which is the most appropriate line of investigation to further investigate a pulmonary embolus?
a CT pulmonary angiogram with lead protection of the patient's abdomen
b Cardiac echo to exclude intracardiac thrombus
c Reduced-dose ventilation/perfusion scan
d MUGA study
e Therapeutic dose heparin till delivery and definitive imaging

29 A journal published details of the ages of a series of 11 patients presenting for lung biopsy. Their ages are listed as 28, 30, 32, 55, 66, 67, 70, 70, 72, 83 and 87.
    What is their median age?
a 60
b 63
c 65
d 67
e 70

30 A 35-year-old female presented to the Emergency Department with acute shortness of breath on a background of progressive exertional dyspnoea and cough over the course of 20 months. She does not smoke. Her initial frontal chest radiograph shows a pneumothorax and a background of a coarse reticulonodular interstitial pattern with multiple cysts in all zones of both lungs. A chest drain tube was inserted and a subsequent CT scan showed numerous diffusely scattered thin-walled cysts surrounded by normal lung parenchyma. A left-sided effusion had a density of –18 HU and the precarinal lymph nodes measured 1.6 cm in short axis. What is the most likely diagnosis?
a Histiocytosis
b Lymphangiomyomatosis
c Emphysema
d Neurofibromatosis
e Bronchiectasis

31 A 32-year-old man developed a low-grade fever and weight loss. He was previously well and had never smoked. CT shows lymphadenopathy on both sides of the diaphragm and a sample taken at mediastinoscopy showed Reed Sternberg cells. There were no further positive findings in the rest of the thorax or abdomen. What is the Ann Arbor stage of this disease?

a Stage I
b Stage II
c Stage III
d Stage IV A
e Stage IV B

32 A 61-year-old female developed gradually worsening hoarseness of her voice. Her PA chest radiograph showed a widened mediastinum and a CT confirmed a lobulated anterior mediastinal mass. The surrounding mediastinal fat showed no stranding fascial planes were preserved. There was no lymphadenopathy and the lungs were of normal appearance. What is the likely density of this lesion?

a Similar to lung
b Similar to mediastinal fat
c Similar to skeletal muscle
d Similar to cancellous bone
e Fluid density

33 A 29-year-old gentleman presented with recurrent right hypochondrial pain and jaundice. He had a peripheral eosinophilia and his chest radiograph showed a cystic structure that contained an air-fluid level with a thin radiolucent crescent in the upper part of the lesion. His Casoni skin test was positive. What is the most likely diagnosis?

a Hamartoma
b *Staphylococcus* abscess
c Aspergillosis
d Hydatid
e Metastatic hepatocellular carcinoma

34 A 75-year-old gentleman who had worked in the construction industry had a chest radiograph prior to an elective cholecystectomy. Multiple calcified pleural plaques were visible bilaterally with basal interstitial shadowing. There was also an ill-defined mass in the left lung. What is the most likely aetiology of the pulmonary tumour?

a Small cell carcinoma
b Bronchoalveolar cell carcinoma
c Squamous cell carcinoma
d Large cell carcinoma
e Aspergilloma

35 A 70-year-old man with long-standing severe rheumatoid arthritis developed progressive dyspnoea. Fine 'Velcro-like' crepitations were audible in his chest and a chest radiograph showed reticulonodular densities and well-circumscribed nodules. Where in the lungs are the reticulonodular densities most likely to be located?

a Apices

b Perihilar

c Subpleural

d Bases

e Paratracheal

36 A 55-year-old man presented with a persistent cough and wheeze. CT of his thorax showed a solitary 2 cm endobronchial polypoidal mass that enhanced vividly in the late arterial phase. There were no other positive findings and a PET scan showed no uptake in this lesion. What is the most likely diagnosis?

a Squamous cell carcinoma

b Rheumatoid nodule

c Carcinoid

d Metastatic nasopharyngeal carcinoma

e Bronchogenic cyst

37 A 78-year-old female patient had a chest radiograph that showed multiple pulmonary nodules of varying sizes in both lungs, without zonal predilection which were thought to be metastases. What is the most likely site of an underlying primary tumour?

a Breast

b Colon

c Bone

d Pancreas

e Ovary

38 A 54-year-old male on long-term methotrexate therapy presented with increasing shortness of breath over several months. Pulmonary function tests demonstrated an obstructive picture and he had no response to a course of antibiotics. A chest radiograph was normal. HRCT reveals mosaic perfusion with air-trapping on expiratory scans, bronchial wall thickening, centrilobular ground-glass and bronchiolectasis. What is the most likely diagnosis?

a Chronic eosinophilic pneumonia

b Bronchiolitis obliterans

c Usual interstitial pneumonia

d Tuberculosis

e Non-specific interstitial pneumonia

39 A four-year-old male presented with a chronic cough. A chest radiograph demonstrated hyperinflation of the lungs with peribronchial thickening and he was treated with a course of antibiotics. Follow-up radiographs demonstrated persistent changes and the development of ring shadows in the right upper lobe. A CT revealed bronchiectasis bilaterally in the upper lobes and bronchoalveolar lavage samples grew *Staphylococcus aureus* and *Pseudomonas aeruginosa*. What is the most likely underlying diagnosis?

a Asthma
b Aspergillosis
c Cystic fibrosis
d Post-infective bronchiectasis
e Tuberculosis

40 In a 74-year-old female with chronic obstructive pulmonary disease (COPD), which of the following descriptions on HRCT would increase the possibility of a *Mycobacterium avium-intracellulare* (MAI) versus *Mycobacterium tuberculosis*?

a Pulmonary consolidation
b Irregular pleural thickening
c Diffuse bronchiectasis and centrilobular nodulation
d Lesions affecting predominantly the apical segments of the lower lobes
e Apical cavitation

41 A 35-year-old female presented with a persistent cough and a chest radiograph was performed. This demonstrated a 2.5-cm mass in the periphery of the right lung and a subsequent CT was performed which confirmed a 2.5-cm lobulated mass in the right lower lobe with a heterogeneous appearance. A focus of low attenuation with the lesion had a density of −100 HU. What is the most appropriate course of action?

a Proceed to a staging abdominal and pelvic CT. The most likely diagnosis is metastatic adenocarcinoma
b Proceed to abdominal CT. The most likely diagnosis is a primary bronchogenic carcinoma
c Advise no further investigations necessary. The most likely diagnosis is a pulmonary hamartoma
d Advise exclusion of granulomatous disease by clinical means
e Advise review of the clinical history for evidence of hydrocarbon inhalation. The most likely diagnosis is lipoid pneumonia

42 A patient with shortness of breath was investigated with a chest radiograph that showed pulmonary infiltrate in a 'reverse bat-wing' distribution. What disease typically has demonstrated this appearance?

a Alveolar proteinosis
b Chronic eosinophilic pneumonia
c Lymphoma

d Goodpasture's syndrome
e Alveolar cell carcinoma

43 A 74-year-old man presented with dyspnoea and chest pain. A chest radiograph showed pleural thickening encasing the right hemithorax and a right pleural effusion. There are no pleural plaques and the visible lung is normal. What is the most likely diagnosis?
a Metastatic thymoma
b Malignant mesothelioma
c Tuberculosis
d Metastatic colonic carcinoma
e Pleural fibroma

44 A 44-year-old male presented with haemoptysis and a chest radiograph was performed. A 1-cm soft-tissue-density nodule was identified projected over the right upper zone. What additional finding is most likely to suggest a malignant aetiology?
a Calcification within the nodule
b Multiple small satellite nodules surrounding the dominant nodule
c Bihilar lymphadenopathy
d Linear densities radiating from the edge of the lesion into the surrounding lung
e The presence of a feeding and draining vessel emanating from the hilar aspect of the nodule

45 A 50-year-old male smoker was investigated for haemoptysis and a bronchocentric 3-cm soft-tissue lesion was seen 1 cm from the carina in the left upper lobe. The maximum visible nodes were 14mm in the left hilum, a 13-mm subcarinal node in the central mediastinum and a 9-mm right hilar node. There was no further parenchymal lesion or effusion and no distant lesions were visible. What is the appropriate TNM staging?
a T2, N1, M0
b T2, N2, M0
c T2, N3, M0
d T3, N2, M0
e T3, N3, M0

46 In a patient with a long-standing history of rheumatoid arthritis, what is the most frequent respiratory manifestation of the disease?
a Pleural effusion
b Diffuse interstitial lung fibrosis
c Multiple well-circumscribed peripheral lung nodules
d Bronchiectasis
e Cardiomegaly

47 A 30-year-old male who had a history of recurrent respiratory infections as a child presented with exertional dyspnoea. On his chest radiograph there is increased transradiancy of the right lung. What additional feature would support a diagnosis of Swyer-James syndrome?
   a Bronchiectasis
   b Mismatched ventilation and perfusion defects on V/Q scan with delayed washout in hyperlucent areas
   c An increase in size of the ipsilateral pulmonary vessels
   d Small contralateral hilum
   e A right-sided aortic knuckle

48 A previously fit and healthy 15-year-old boy presents to his GP with an expiratory wheeze. The chest radiograph is normal. What is the most likely diagnosis?
   a Tracheal hamartoma
   b Bronchogenic cyst
   c Tracheobronchopathia osteoplastica
   d Asthma
   e Endobronchial carcinoid

49 A 56-year-old female with a history of breast carcinoma presented with chest pain that was atypical for cardiac pain and she was afebrile. A chest radiograph demonstrated right upper lobe opacification adjacent to the mediastinum with a very well-defined lateral border and elevation of the right hilum. What is the most likely explanation for these findings?
   a Right upper lobe pneumonia
   b Lymphangitis carcinomatosis
   c Scleroderma
   d Radiation pneumonitis
   e Chemotherapy-induced lung disease

50 A 26-year-old Afro-Caribbean lady presented with a painful rash on her shins, arthralgia, fever and malaise. A frontal CXR demonstrated bi-hilar lymphadenopathy, but no parenchymal abnormality. What is the most likely diagnosis?
   a Primary pulmonary TB
   b Lymphoma
   c PCP pneumonia
   d Post-primary TB
   e Sarcoidosis

51 A patient underwent an HRCT that demonstrated small lung volumes and coarsened septal thickening in a predominantly subpleural and basal distribution. There were areas of honeycombing and traction bronchiectasis and bronchiolectasis. What is the most likely diagnosis?

a Radiation fibrosis
b Silicosis
c Chronic extrinsic allergic alveolitis (hypersensitivity pneumonitis)
d Usual interstitial pneumonia (UIP)
e Beryliosis

52 A 62-year-old patient with ongoing dyspnoea underwent CT of the chest. Among other findings it demonstrated two ill-defined foci of consolidation within the posterior and apical segments of the right upper lobe. In addition, within the remainder of the right lung, and to a lesser extent the left lung, there was a more diffuse abnormality characterised by small (<4mm) centrilobular, well-defined nodules within 1 cm of the pleural surface. These nodules were connected by linear, branching opacities. What is the most likely cause for these findings?
a Obliterative bronchiolitis
b Primary pulmonary lymphoma
c Respiratory syncytial virus infection
d Reactivation tuberculosis
e Renal cell carcinoma metastases

53 A 34-year-old banker presented with dyspnoea on exertion and intermittent chest pain. She was slightly cyanosed and mildly hypoxic at rest, becoming more so on standing. A chest radiograph demonstrated a lobulated 3-cm mass in the left lower zone with a small, rounded focus of calcification within it. 'Cordlike' bands are seen extending from the mass to the left hilum. What is the most likely diagnosis?
a Melanoma metastasis
b Pulmonary capillary haemangiomatosis
c Pulmonary hamartoma
d Angiomyolipoma
e Pulmonary arteriovenous malformation

54 A 43-year-old social worker underwent chest radiography and chest CT. On the chest radiograph there was right-sided widening of the mediastinum in the region of the right hilum and calcification was also seen within the mediastinum with signs of right heart dilatation. Within the right lung there was peribronchial cuffing, septal thickening and wedges of consolidation. CT confirms the presence of a focal, partly calcified right perihilar mediastinal mass, right heart dilatation and peripheral wedge shaped areas of consolidation in the right lung. What is the most likely diagnosis?
a Fibrosing mediastinitis
b Mediastinal granuloma
c Primary pulmonary lymphoma
d Thymic carcinoma
e Histoplasmosis

55 A 56-year-old airport baggage handler presented to the respiratory clinic with dyspnoea and cough in addition to weight loss and occasional chest pain. He had smoked 60 cigarettes a day for over 30 years. There was no evidence of finger clubbing on examination and pulmonary function tests demonstrated a mixed obstructive-restrictive pattern with reduced diffusion capacity. Ground-glass opacification, air trapping, centrilobular nodules and mild septal thickening were seen on HRCT. What is the most likely diagnosis?

a Usual interstitial pneumonitis (UIP)
b Respiratory bronchiolitis-associated interstitial lung disease (RBILD)
c Lymphocytic interstitial pneumonitis (LIP)
d Non-specific interstitial pneumonitis (NSIP)
e Cryptogenic organising pneumonia (COP)

56 HRCT was performed on a 60-year-old patient who had a long history of dyspnoea. He was no longer able to climb the stairs at home due to breathlessness. His chest radiograph showed changes of fibrosis. What further finding on HRCT would most favour a diagnosis of sarcoid over chronic extrinsic allergic alveolitis (EAA)?

a Interstitial thickening
b Traction bronchiectasis
c Air trapping
d Pleural effusions
e Nodular thickening of the fissures

57 A 52-year-old miner presented with increasing exertional dyspnoea and cough, which were becoming more severe over many years. Fine mid- and upper-zone inspiratory crepitations were apparent on examination. His chest radiograph showed small (<10 mm), rounded mid- and upper-zone opacities some of which displayed central calcification. There was also a reticular mid- and upper-zone pattern of opacification. HRCT confirms the presence of thickened intra- and interlobular septal lines and nodules with some thicker parenchymal fibrotic bands and traction bronchiectasis. There is bilateral mediastinal adenopathy with peripheral eggshell calcification. What is the likely diagnosis?

a Silicosis
b Coal workers pneumoconiosis
c Siderosis
d Stannosis
e Caplan's syndrome

58 A 54-year-old female presented to the ENT Department with shortness of breath and increasing stridor. She had a history of chronic myeloid leukaemia and during a recent course of chemotherapy suffered from severe pneumonia and was admitted to ITU for support. CT demonstrated a short, concentric stenosis within the mid to distal trachea. What is the most likely explanation for these findings?

a Post-intubation stricture
b Secondary amyloidosis of the trachea
c Post-pneumonic stricture
d Squamous cell carcinoma of the trachea
e Tracheobronchopathia osteochondroplastica

59 A 32-year-old flight attendant presented with shortness of breath, fever, cough and haemoptysis. There were bilateral crepitations on auscultation and several blue/red raised skin lesions were noted. His CD4 lymphocyte count is 120 (normal >500). HRCT of the chest demonstrated patches of numerous, ill-defined nodules in a perihilar distribution and septal thickening. There was moderate hilar lymphadenopathy but no pleural effusion. What is the most likely diagnosis?
a *Streptococcus* pneumonia
b *Pneumocystis carinii* pneumonia
c Kaposi's sarcoma
d *Mycobacterium avium-intracellulare* infection
e AIDS-related lymphoma of B-cell origin

60 A 40-year-old homeless man presented to the Emergency Department with dyspnoea, fever and cough. Crepitations and bronchial breathing were heard on auscultation. Blood analysis revealed a neutrophilia, macrocytic anaemia and high gamma-glutamyl transpeptidase and alkaline phosphatase. There was bilateral patchy airspace opacification on his chest radiograph and CT demonstrated moderate upper zone centrilobular emphysema with consolidation within the posterior segments of both upper lobes and middle and right lower lobes. What is the most likely diagnosis?
a *Mycoplasma* pneumonia
b Primary tuberculosis
c Aspiration pneumonia
d Streptococcal pneumonia
e Invasive aspergillosis

61 A 47-year-old shop assistant presented with a long history of allergic rhinitis and asthma. In the previous few weeks she had also experienced increasing dyspnoea, arthralgia and diarrhoea, which was occasionally blood stained. Blood analysis showed an elevated eosinophil count, mild renal impairment and positive pANCA antibody. There was patchy, non-segmental, bilateral airspace opacification on HRCT with small nodules. What is the most likely unifying diagnosis?
a Wegener's granulomatosis
b Goodpasture's disease
c Histoplasmosis
d Polyarteritis nodosa
e Churg-Strauss disease

62 A 47-year-old male patient became markedly hypoxic 24 hours after bilateral lung transplantation for idiopathic pulmonary fibrosis. The patient did not have any other significant medical history. He had not been extubated due to increasing oxygen demands over the preceding hours and his chest radiograph showed perihilar airspace opacification and bibasal pleural effusions. He was afebrile and was not fluid overloaded. What is the most likely diagnosis?
    a Reperfusion syndrome
    b Cardiogenic pulmonary oedema
    c Acute transplant rejection
    d Post-transplant lymphoproliferative disease
    e Post-transplantation infection

63 A patient is due for an angiographic examination but is concerned due to a previous complication following angiography. On his previous admission he developed a femoral pseudoaneurysm (false femoral aneurysm) which required surgical exploration. He asks you how likely this is to happen again. What would make another false femoral pseudoaneurysm more likely?
    a Catheterisation of the common femoral artery
    b Diagnostic angiography
    c High femoral puncture
    d Obesity
    e Overly vigorous post-procedure compression

64 A cardiology inpatient underwent an ultrasound examination of the groin that showed a 5-cm lesion immediately superficial to the proximal superficial femoral artery. On colour duplex this lesion demonstrated turbulent flow. There was no evidence of communication with the venous system. There was no evidence of infection. What is the most appropriate treatment?
    a Observation and routine ultrasound at four weeks
    b Application of a manual compression device
    c Ultrasound-guided compression
    d Percutaneous thrombin injection
    e Surgical exploration

65 An 82-year-old female patient was undergoing a percutaneous transhepatic cholangiogram and biliary stent insertion to relieve jaundice related to a hilar cholangiocarcinoma. She was anxious and found the procedure painful so was given several intravenous boluses of midazolam and fentanyl during the procedure. After 45 minutes she had received a total of 12 mg of midazolam. Her respiratory rate was noted to be low and she became less responsive. What is the most appropriate flumazenil regime in this situation?
    a 200 mg IV bolus over 15 seconds followed by 100 mg at 1-minute intervals up to a maximum of 1000 mg
    b 500 mg IV bolus over 15 seconds followed by 250 mg at 1-minute intervals up to a maximum of 5000 mg

c 1000 mg bolus

d 100–400 mg/hr infusion

e 1000–4000 mg/hr infusion

66 A 74-year-old man was being investigated by a cardiologist for repeated episodes of 'flash' pulmonary oedema. He was hypertensive and echocardiography showed good left ventricular function. Renal artery Doppler and subsequent MR angiography confirmed severe bilateral renal artery stenosis. He was known to have benign prostatic hypertrophy, but there was no renal collecting system dilatation on ultrasound. Following extensive discussion, the decision was made to attempt bilateral renal artery stenting. What benefit over optimal medical therapy is this most likely to result in?

a Improve hypertension

b Improve renal function

c Improve symptoms of prostatism

d Reduce episodes of pulmonary oedema

e Reduce mortality

67 A 42-year-old woman with symptoms of dyspareunia and dysmenorrhoea was found to have bulky uterine fibroids on ultrasound. Following discussion with her gynaecologist she was referred for uterine artery embolisation. During the embolisation procedure it is noted that a significant degree of the fibroid blood supply is derived from the ovarian artery. With the aim of temporarily occluding the ovarian artery, what embolic agent is most appropriate?

a Cyanoacrylate (glue)

b Ethyl alcohol

c Gelfoam

d Polyvinyl alcohol

e Steel coils

68 A 53-year-old alcoholic was admitted with oesophageal variceal bleeding and decompensated alcoholic liver disease. Repeated endoscopy with attempted sclerotherapy and banding was unsuccessful in resolving the bleeding and a transjugular intrahepatic portosystemic shunt (TIPS) procedure was considered. What would be an absolute contraindication to TIPS?

a Ascites

b Budd-Chiari syndrome

c Hepatic encephalopathy

d Hepatic failure

e Severe right-sided heart failure

69 A patient with severe hypertension refractory to maximal medical therapy had a renal angiogram. What angiographic features would suggest that percutaneous transluminal angioplasty (PTA) would be beneficial?
  a Mid-renal artery stenosis
  b Multiple intra-renal aneurysms
  c Ostial stenosis
  d Small diameter renal arteries
  e String-of-beads appearance

70 You are undertaking a lower limb angiogram in a patient with an acutely ischaemic limb and are considering using intra-arterial thrombolysis. In which of the following situations would you be happy to administer rtPA?
  a The patient underwent cardiopulmonary resuscitation one week ago
  b The patient is known to have cerebral metastases
  c The patient reported an episode of haematemesis
  d The patient is pregnant
  e The patient received streptokinase 10 years ago

Cardiothoracic and vascular radiology

PAPER 3

1   A cyanotic neonate has a chest radiograph that shows pulmonary plethora
    and cardiomegaly. What additional finding on the chest radiograph is most
    suggestive of a diagnosis of transposition of the great vessels?
    a   Cardiomegaly at birth
    b   An enlarged aortic arch
    c   Global cardiac enlargement
    d   An enlarged pulmonary trunk
    e   A narrowed superior mediastinum

2   A two-month-old baby presented with increasing dyspnoea and cyanosis.
    A chest radiograph revealed a marked reduction in the pulmonary vasculature
    and an absent aortic knuckle. The heart was not enlarged. What is the most
    likely diagnosis?
    a   Ventricular septal defect
    b   Tetralogy of Fallot
    c   Truncus arteriosus
    d   Total anomalous pulmonary venous drainage
    e   Ebstein's anomaly

3   A 56-year-old man had a chest radiograph following several episodes of chest
    pain. This showed a soft tissue-density lesion in the left cardiophrenic angle
    that has an acute angle with the diaphragm. A CT was performed which
    showed this to be a well-defined mass with an average Hounsfield unit value
    of 25. Magnetic resonance imaging (MRI) was also performed as part of his
    chest pain work-up and the mass was of low signal on T1-weighted imaging.
    What is the most likely diagnosis?
    a   A cardiophrenic fat pad
    b   A lung sequestration
    c   A pericardial lipoma
    d   A pericardial cyst
    e   A lymph node

4 A 46-year-old female presented to the Emergency Department in heart failure with a history of chest pain. A chest radiograph demonstrated an enlarged heart and bilateral pleural effusions. What imaging finding would suggest a diagnosis of constrictive pericarditis rather than restrictive cardiomyopathy?

a A pericardial thickness on CT of 4 mm
b Dilated right atrium
c Ascites
d Absence of ventricular hypertrophy
e Global subendocardial late gadolinium enhancement on MRI

5 A patient was due to have an aortic stent graft. The native artery measured 28–30 mm in diameter. What diameter of stent would be most appropriate?

a 25 mm
b 28 mm
c 30 mm
d 33 mm
e 36 mm

6 A 45-year-old male with known ischaemic heart disease presented with increasing shortness of breath on exertion and peripheral oedema. Echocardiography showed impaired left ventricular function. A cardiac magnetic resonance study was performed. What finding would be most consistent with hibernating myocardium?

a 75% Subendocardial delayed enhancement
b Normal myocardial contractility at rest
c No myocardial delayed enhancement
d Epicardial hyperenhancement
e Patchy hyperenhancement of myocardium

7 A one-year-old male presented to the Emergency Department following a syncopal episode. On clinical examination there was an audible murmur and the child subsequently had an echocardiogram, which demonstrated a solid echogenic mass closely applied to the right ventricular wall. What is the most likely diagnosis?

a Teratoma
b Myxoma
c Rhabdomyoma
d Angioma
e Lymphoma

8 A 43-year-old female presented with fatigue and dyspnoea to her GP who requested a chest radiograph. This showed an enlarged heart and pulmonary outflow tracts with a small aorta and pulmonary plethora. What is the most likely cardiac abnormality to explain this appearance?

a Ventricular septal defect
b Atrial septal defect
c Aortic regurgitation
d Pulmonary stenosis
e Ebstein's anomaly

9 A neonate presented with cyanosis. Their chest radiograph revealed cardiomegaly and diminished pulmonary blood flow. What is the most likely diagnosis?
a Pulmonary stenosis
b Truncus arteriosus
c A ventricular septal defect
d Transposition of the great vessels
e Tetralogy of Fallot

10 A 27-year-old male presented to the Emergency Department following a road traffic accident. He was haemodynamically unstable and complained of severe chest pain. His initial supine chest radiograph was normal and abdominal examination was also unremarkable. A CT thorax was requested to investigate possible aortic injury. What is the most likely finding on CT of an aortic transection?
a A contour deformity on the inner aortic wall at the level of the isthmus
b Increased density within the superior mediastinum
c Pericardial effusion
d Contrast extravasation from the aorta at the level of the diaphragmatic hiatus
e Occlusion of the subclavian artery

11 A 68-year-old male presented to the Emergency Department with shortness of breath. A chest radiograph revealed a pacemaker box lying within the left pectoral pocket with three leads arising from it. The first two leads lie within the right atrial appendage and right ventricle and the distal tip of the third lead is projected over the left ventricle. In which structure is the third lead most likely to be positioned?
a Interventricular septum
b Epicardium
c Coronary sinus
d Cardiac vein
e Persistent left superior vena cava

12 A 24-year-old female was investigated for syncopal episodes. A 24-hour ECG was normal and a coronary angiogram was suspicious for anomalous coronary artery anatomy. A gated coronary artery CT was requested. What arterial course is most likely to cause haemodynamic compromise and therefore require intervention?

   a Right coronary artery arising from the left coronary sinus and passing anterior to the aorta

   b Right coronary artery arising from the left coronary sinus and passing posterior to the aorta

   c Circumflex artery arising from the right coronary sinus passing posterior

   d Circumflex artery arising from the left coronary artery and passing into the atrioventricular groove

   e Left main stem arising from the non-coronary sinus and passing anteriorly

13 A 46-year-old Russian sailor presented with malaise and chest pain. In the course of the investigations he underwent CT scanning of his chest and abdomen. His VDRL and MHA-TP (for *Treponema pallidum*) tests are positive. What is the most likely finding on his CT?

   a Saccular aneurysm of the ascending aorta with thin, dystrophic wall calcification

   b Saccular aneurysm of the ascending aorta with interrupted calcification, para-aortic gas collection and adjacent reactive lymph node enlargement

   c Fusiform aneurysm of the descending aorta with cresenteric mural thrombus. There is ectasia of the remainder of the aorta with heavy atherosclerosis

   d Fusiform aneurysm of the abdominal aorta demonstrating mural thickening and extensive surrounding fibrosis

   e Fusiform aneurysm of the descending aorta with an irregular wall and active extravasations of intravenous contrast

14 A 23-year-old professional footballer presents with shortness of breath disproportionate to the level of exertion. He has not experienced any chest pain and on further questioning he states that his brother died suddenly at school during an athletics match. He has never known his father, but his mother is in good health. What imaging finding most suggests a diagnosis of hypertrophic cardiomyopathy (HCM) over arrythmogenic right ventricular dysplasia (ARVD):

   a Fibro-fatty infiltration of the right ventricular wall

   b Segmental right ventricular wall motion abnormality

   c Right ventricular aneurysm

   d Aortic root dilatation

   e Left ventricular outflow narrowing

15 A 59-year-old truck driver presented with severe chest pain and dyspnoea. His ECG demonstrated ST segment elevation in leads V4–V6 and on biochemical analysis troponin levels were elevated. Following several days' stay in hospital he was discharged. On review at six weeks echocardiography demonstrates an akinetic portion of the left ventricular wall and delayed enhancement cardiac MR images demonstrate high signal at 10 minutes in same area of the left ventricular wall. What is the most likely explanation for these imaging findings?

a LV aneurysm
b 'Stunned' myocardium
c Focal myocarditis
d Focal myocardial fibrosis
e 'Hibernating' myocardium

16 A middle-aged gentleman complained of frequent throbbing headaches and cramping of his lower limbs after moderate exertion. He was investigated and a CT of his thorax showed a narrowing at the junction of the aortic arch and descending aorta. Rib notching was visible on his chest radiograph. Which ribs are likely to be most severely affected?

a Superior border first to sixth ribs
b Superior border second and third ribs
c Inferior border third and fourth ribs
d Superior border seventh to ninth ribs
e Inferior border sixth to eighth ribs

17 The pre-employment chest radiograph of an asymptomatic 32-year-old female shows mild pulmonary plethora. Subsequent investigation with a CT thorax reveals abnormal venous drainage of the right upper lobe. Where is this lobe most likely to drain?

a Right atrium
b Superior vena cava
c Suprahepatic portion of the inferior vena cava
d Coronary sinus
e Portal vein

18 A 32-year-old intravenous drug user was admitted for management of a brain abscess. His medical records showed recurrent admissions with life-threatening epistaxis. Physical examination revealed multiple vascular blemishes on his lips, palate, conjunctiva and fingers. On chest auscultation, there was a bruit in the right lung base and a chest radiograph was performed. This showed a serpiginous mass in the right lower zone. What is the most likely underlying diagnosis?

a Sickle cell disease
b Factor V deficiency
c AIDS
d Hereditary haemorrhagic telangiectasia
e Vitamin K deficiency

19 A 60-year-old diabetic gentleman with hypertension and hyperlipidaemia presented with sudden onset intractable chest pain radiating to his jaw and back. The initial working diagnosis was an acute myocardial event and a chest radiograph was performed as part of the work-up. This showed a widened mediastinum and an urgent CT aortogram was arranged. This demonstrated a dissection of the ascending aorta, which extended into the arch and distally into the first portion of the descending aorta. What would be the next most appropriate step in management?

a Confirm the diagnosis with TOE (trans-oesophageal echocardiogram)
b Reduce the peak systolic blood pressure to <120 mmHg
c Perform serial monitoring with TOE to determine progression
d Immediate surgery
e No intervention is necessary

20 A 65-year-old woman with a history of an inferior myocardial infarction nine months previously underwent a cardiac MRI. When would you expect peak enhancement of the myocardium in the left ventricular free wall following administration of gadolinium-based contrast?

a No enhancement will occur
b Within 10 seconds
c 20–30 seconds
d 5–7 minutes
e 10–15 minutes

21 A 45-year-old gentleman presented with dyspnoea on exertion and was found to have a cardiac murmur. Echocardiography showed an atrial mass with internal Doppler signal. Where in the atrial cavity is this mass most likely to arise from?

a Left atrial appendage
b Attached by a thin stalk to the left side of the inter-atrial septum
c Broad based on the right side of the inter-atrial septum
d Bi-lobed appearance in both atria arising from both sides of the inter-atrial septum
e On the atrial aspect of the mitral valve

22 A 23-year-old male was involved in a high-speed motor vehicle accident. He complained of severe chest pain and was haemodynamically unstable. The working diagnosis was that of a traumatic aortic rupture and he was transferred immediately to theatre. Where in the thoracic aorta is the rupture most likely?

a Ascending aorta, just distal to the aortic valve
b Ascending aorta, just prior to the origin of the right brachiocephalic trunk
c Aortic arch
d Aortic isthmus, just distal to the left subclavian artery
e Descending aorta, at the level of the diaphragmatic hiatus

23 A 56-year-old gentleman had a chest radiograph as part of an application for a working visa. This showed a widened mediastinum, which was subsequently shown to be due to a focal dilatation of the thoracic aorta and he tested positive for *Treponema pallidum*. Which part of the aorta is most likely to be affected?

a Aortic valve

b Aortic sinus

c Aortic arch

d Proximal descending aorta

e Distal descending thoracic aorta immediately above diaphragm

24 A 72-year-old gentleman with long-standing atrial fibrillation experienced several episodes of transient neurological deficits. An echocardiogram was performed as part of his work-up and an echogenic mass was seen that did not show any internal Doppler signal. Where is this mass most likely to be?

a Atrial side of the tricuspid valve

b Left ventricle, on the interventricular septum

c Right atrium, on the inter-atrial septum

d Left atrial appendage

e Pulmonary valve

25 A patient suffering from type 1 diabetes underwent a whole body PET CT for the staging of cancer. What is the most appropriate advice to optimise the quality of their scan?

a Caffeine should be avoided as it can increase or decrease cardiac FDG uptake

b Blood sugar should be below 3 mg/L

c The patient should be nil by mouth for 24 hours

d The patient can be given 2–5 u insulin immediately prior to FDG injection

e Uptake in smooth muscle should be ignored if the haemoglobin A1c (HbA1c) level is higher than expected

26 A 34-year-old fit and well female presented with a two-week history of right-sided pleuritic chest pain and tenderness following a recent chest infection, which had cleared after treatment with antibiotics. She is not short of breath. A bone scan showed a solitary focus of Tc-99m-labelled MDP uptake in the region of the lateral tenth right rib and no other abnormalities. What is the most likely explanation for these findings?

a Pulmonary infarct from pulmonary embolus

b Solitary metastasis from an occult primary

c Cough fracture

d Costochondritis

e Residual infection

27 A 100-kg male patient underwent a cardiac rest and stress Myoview study to assess for reversible coronary arterial disease. The images showed reduced uptake in the inferior cardiac wall on both the rest and stress images. He tolerated the study well but experienced dizziness and a mild drop in his blood pressure during the stress phase. What is the likely cause for the appearances on the study?

   a Reversible ischaemia in the inferior wall – right coronary artery territory

   b Irreversible loss of cardiac viability in the left anterior descending territory

   c High-sitting diaphragm causing artefact

   d Reversible ischaemia in the left circumflex territory

   e Cardiac hibernation in the left anterior descending distribution

28 A 42-year-old woman presented after a long-haul flight with shortness of breath, hypoxia, tachycardia, new right bundle branch block on her ECG and pleuritic chest pain. No coexistent cardiopulmonary pathology is present. A chest radiograph taken 36 hours ago shows no abnormality. What is the next appropriate step according to the guidelines laid out by the British Thoracic Society?

   a CT pulmonary angiography

   b Ventilation/perfusion scan (V/Q)

   c D dimer blood test

   d Repeat chest radiograph

   e Conventional pulmonary angiography

29 A two-year-old child underwent a palliative procedure for a cyanotic congenital heart abnormality. A post-operative CT demonstrated a poly-tetrafluoroethylene (PTFE) graft between the subclavian artery and the ipsilateral branch of the pulmonary artery. What surgical procedure has been performed?

   a Blalock-Hanlon procedure

   b Glenn procedure

   c Rashkind procedure

   d Norwood procedure

   e Blalock-Taussig shunt

30 A pre-employment screening chest radiograph on a 40-year-old female revealed a solitary mass in the periphery of the right upper zone. This was of fat density and 'popcorn' calcification was visible. The radiograph was otherwise normal and the patient was asymptomatic. What is the most likely diagnosis?

   a Pancoast tumour

   b Pulmonary hamartoma

   c Tuberculoma

   d Pulmonary nocardia

   e Sarcoid

31 A 32-year-old man developed a low-grade fever and weight loss and was found to have Hodgkin's lymphoma with lymphadenopathy in both thorax and abdomen. Involvement of which extra-nodal site is associated with the worst prognosis?

a Pleural effusion

b Spleen

c Thymus

d Bone

e Small intestine

32 A 70-year-old gentleman suffered from shortness of breath following a total hip replacement and a ventilation/perfusion scan was performed, which showed a mismatched perfusion defect. What is the most likely cause?

a Emphysema

b Pulmonary hypertension

c Fat embolism

d Pleural effusion

e Lung collapse

33 A 29-year-old gentleman presented with recurrent pain and jaundice. He had a peripheral eosinophilia and his chest radiograph showed a cystic structure that contained an air-fluid level with a thin radiolucent crescent in the upper part of the lesion. His Casoni skin test was positive. Where is this lesion most likely to be located within the lungs?

a Left apex

b Right lower lobe

c Perihilar region

d Within a fissure

e Peribronchial

34 An 18-year-old female with recurrent chest infections and left-sided chest pain was investigated and found to have an 8-cm smooth oval mass in the left lower zone on her chest radiograph. Further investigation with CT shows multiple air-filled thin-walled cysts, which did not communicate with the bronchial tree. The mass enhances at the same time as the thoracic aorta. Where is the venous drainage of the mass most likely to lead?

a Pulmonary veins

b Azygos vein

c Superior vena cava

d Intercostal veins

e Coronary veins

35 An elderly male patient with long-standing severe rheumatoid arthritis
    developed progressive dyspnoea and a chest radiograph showed multiple
    nodules on a background of coarse reticulonodular densities. Where in the
    lungs are the pulmonary nodules most likely to be located?
    a Lung periphery
    b Perihilar
    c Paratracheal
    d Along the fissures
    e No predilection for any lung zones

36 A 55-year-old man presented with a persistent cough and wheeze. CT of his
    thorax showed a solitary 2-cm endobronchial polypoidal mass that enhanced
    vividly in the late arterial phase. There were no other positive findings and
    a PET scan showed no uptake in this lesion. From which artery is the blood
    supply to this lesion most likely to be derived?
    a Pulmonary artery
    b Bronchial artery
    c Adjacent intercostal artery
    d Internal mammary artery
    e Inferior thyroid artery

37 Following radiotherapy for thoracic Hodgkin's disease, a new anterior medi-
    astinal cystic structure was identified on CT thorax of a young adult male. It
    was well defined and showed no aggressive features. What is the most likely
    diagnosis?
    a Bronchogenic cyst
    b Thymic cyst
    c Pericardial cyst
    d Oesophageal enteric cyst
    e Pancreatic pseudocyst tracking up into the mediastinum

38 A 20-year-old man presented with his fifth episode of pneumonia in two
    years. A chest radiograph revealed an abnormal density behind the left car-
    diac shadow and consolidation distal to this lesion. A CT was performed,
    which showed a soft-tissue mass with a feeding vessel from the thoracic aorta.
    What is the most likely diagnosis?
    a Bronchopulmonary sequestration
    b Bronchogenic cyst
    c Cystic adenomatoid malformation
    d An anomalous left pulmonary artery
    e Arteriovenous malformation

39 A previously fit and well 56-year-old female presented with a two-day history
    of chest pain, pyrexia and productive cough. She had a neutrophilia and her
    PA and lateral chest radiographs demonstrated a 4-cm round mass in the left
    lower lobe. What is the most likely causative organism?

a *Staphylococcus aureus*
b *Streptococcus pneumoniae*
c *Mycobacterium tuberculosis*
d *Streptococcus pyogenes*
e *Klebsiella*

40 A 65-year-old male returned from travelling abroad in South America and presented with fever, cough and malaise. A chest radiograph demonstrated non-specific subsegmental infiltrates. The patient recovered with no medical intervention and a repeat chest radiograph obtained a year later as part of a visa application showed multiple punctate calcifications. What is the most likely diagnosis?
a Tuberculosis
b Histoplasmosis
c Coccidioidomycosis
d Blastomycosis
e Sarcoidosis

41 A 30-year-old male smoker presented with a non-productive cough, weight loss and dyspnoea. His chest radiograph showed a diffuse, ill-defined reticulonodular pattern with preserved lung volumes. The cardiomediastinal contours and hilar were normal. On HRCT there are thin-walled cysts <5 mm in size and centrilobular nodules with normal intervening lung. What is the most likely diagnosis?
a Sarcoidosis
b Langerhans cell histiocytosis (LCH)
c Idiopathic pulmonary fibrosis
d Lymphangiomyomatosis (LAM)
e Emphysema

42 A 69-year-old female smoker presented with dyspnoea and weight loss. A chest radiograph showed reticular densities, Kerley lines and hilar lymphadenopathy with a normal heart size. Interlobular septal thickening with nodular pattern and a right-sided pleural effusion were visible on a subsequent CT. What is the most likely diagnosis?
a Usual interstitial pneumonia
b Sarcoidosis
c Lymphangitis carcinomatosis
d Lymphoid interstitial pneumonia
e Left ventricular failure

43 An 18-year-old male was investigated for lethargy and haemoptysis. A chest radiograph revealed multiple lung nodules, which contained small irregular calcifications. Assuming these lesions to be metastases, what it the most likely underlying primary tumour?

a Pancreas

b Renal

c Prostate

d Testis

e Lung

44 A 56-year-old female with cough and dyspnoea was noted to have a calcified lung nodule on chest radiography. What pattern of calcification would make malignancy more likely?

a Completely calcified lesion

b Multiple small foci of calcification

c Concentric calcification

d Central calcification

e Popcorn calcification

45 A 45-year-old man presented to the Emergency Department with severe dyspnoea, pleuritic chest pain, malaise and diarrhoea. Blood tests showed hyponatraemia and a chest radiograph showed a moderate-sized pleural effusion, unilateral pulmonary infiltrates and prominent lymphadenopathy. In view of a recent local outbreak of Legionnaires' disease at a local conference centre this diagnosis was considered. What finding in the work-up would make a different diagnosis more likely?

a Prominent lymphadenopathy

b A moderate pleural effusion

c Unilateral pulmonary infiltrates

d Hyponatraemia

e Pleuritic chest pain

46 A 46-year-old female presented with a vague history of dyspnoea and chest pain. A chest radiograph demonstrated nonspecific findings of atelectasis, a small right-sided pleural effusion and patchy infiltrates. A CT pulmonary angiogram showed thrombus within the pulmonary arteries. What additional finding would be most suggestive of chronic rather than acute thromboembolic disease?

a A large volume of disease

b The presence of systemic hypertension

c Narrowing of the peripheral pulmonary vessels

d Enlargement of the pulmonary arteries

e Centrally placed thrombus

47 A 24-year-old fit and well man had an occupational chest radiograph that showed loss of the right heart border and a straight left heart border. What is the most likely diagnosis?
a Pectus excavatum
b Middle lobe consolidation
c Right lower lobe collapse
d Right atrial enlargement
e Oesophageal dilatation

48 On chest radiography, which of the following features is more in keeping with a diagnosis of bronchiectasis than bronchiolitis?
a Bronchial wall thickening
b Bronchial dilatation
c Atelectasis
d Tiny nodules
e Lobar consolidation

49 A 30-year-old male smoker presented to the Respiratory Clinic with dyspnoea and a productive cough. Spirometry demonstrated reduced lung function and the chest radiograph hyperinflation and bi-basal bullae formation with relative sparing of the upper zones. What is the most likely diagnosis?
a Early onset chronic obstructive pulmonary disease (COPD)
b Langerhans cell histiocytosis
c Congenital lobar emphysema
d α 1 antitrypsin deficiency
e Lymphangioleiomyomatosis (LAM)

50 You are asked to review a chest radiograph by a respiratory physician. There is a discrete mass arising behind the heart on the left. The lateral border is smooth and rounded. Medially, the mass obscures the lateral border of the descending thoracic aorta. No other abnormalities are visible. What is the most likely diagnosis?
a Thyroid carcinoma
b Schwannoma
c Teratoma
d Ectopic parathyroid adenoma
e Lymphoma

51 A 24-year-old primary school teacher presents to the acute medical unit with right-sided pleuritic chest pain and dyspnoea. She has never been unwell and takes no regular medication except the combined oral contraceptive pill. Examination is unremarkable except for tachypnoea and her oxygen saturations are 92% on air. She refused arterial blood gas analysis. Her chest radiograph demonstrated right mid-zone opacification and a ventilation/perfusion scan was arranged. What appearance would be most compatible with a diagnosis of pulmonary thromboembolism?

a Segmental perfusion defect much larger than an associated ventilation defect

b Sub-segmental matched ventilation/perfusion defect

c Non-segmental matched ventilation/perfusion defect

d Non-segmental mismatched perfusion defect

e Segmental matched ventilation/perfusion defect

52 A patient with known hypersensitivity pneumonitis (extrinsic allergic alveolitis) underwent HRCT of the chest after presenting to the Respiratory Clinic with increasing dyspnoea. During the last part of the scan a medical student asks you why the radiographer has scanned the patient prone on expiration. What is the most rational explanation?

a A functional test to see how mobile the patient is and how long they can exhale and hold their breath

b To accentuate differential lung attenuation caused by air trapping and obviate any gravitational (dependent) changes seen on the supine scan

c To obviate any gravitational (dependent) changes seen on the supine scan and reduce differential lung attenuation caused by air trapping

d To accentuate gravitational (dependent) changes and accentuate differential lung attenuation caused by air trapping

e To reduce differential lung attenuation caused by air trapping and accentuate gravitational (dependent) changes

53 A 47-year-old primary school teacher, due to emigrate to Australia, underwent chest radiography that showed a mass in the superior mediastinum. The mass extended into the neck and there was slight deviation of the trachea to the left. No information is available as to whether the patient has any symptoms or signs. What is the most likely cause for this appearance?

a Mediastinal dermoid

b Thyroid enlargement

c Thymic tumour

d Lymphadenopathy

e Fibrosing mediastinitis

54 A 12-year-old boy with a long-standing history of mild dysphagia underwent endoscopy, which demonstrated extrinsic compression of the mid oesophagus. The paediatric team were keen to avoid radiation exposure and the patient was re-booked for endoscopic ultrasound. This showed a rounded,

thin-walled, echo-poor cyst located anterior to the oesophagus in a subcarinal location. Mucoid material was aspirated from the cyst. What is the most likely diagnosis?

a Extralobar pulmonary sequestration
b Thymic cyst
c Intralobar pulmonary sequestration
d Tarlov cyst
e Bronchogenic cyst

55 A 50-year-old laboratory technician presented acutely with severe dyspnoea. She gave a history of recent upper respiratory tract infection and examination revealed cyanosis, tachypnoea and bilateral widespread crepitations. Pulmonary function tests showed a restrictive pattern with reduced diffusing capacity. Several days after admission her oxygen requirements increased and required non-invasive ventilatory support. A repeat chest radiograph showed bilateral patchy airspace opacification with air bronchograms sparing the costophrenic angles. HRCT showed consolidation and ground-glass change, bronchial dilatation and architectural distortion and subsequent lung biopsy demonstrated hyaline membrane formation. What is the most likely diagnosis?

a Acute interstitial pneumonitis (AIP)
b Cryptogenic organising pneumonitis (COP)
c *Mycoplasma avium* infection
d Hypersensitivity pneumonitis
e Respiratory bronchiolitis-associated interstitial lung disease (RBILD)

56 A 72-year-old retired policeman, with a known history of cardiac arrhythmias and increasing dyspnoea over six months, presented acutely with worsening breathlessness. HRCT showed septal thickening and diffuse ground-glass changes in a largely symmetrical and predominantly basal distribution. The liver was also markedly more dense than the spleen. What is the most likely explanation for his dyspnoea?

a Right heart failure
b Drug-induced pulmonary damage
c Usual interstitial pneumonitis (UIP)
d Legionella pneumonia
e Primary pulmonary lymphoma

57 A patient with advanced acute myeloid leukaemia became acutely breathless following a large blood transfusion. He was markedly tachypnoeic at rest and blood gas analysis revealed type 1 respiratory failure. His coagulation screen showed a prolonged activated thromboplastin time and the fibrinogen level was markedly reduced. The on-call haematologist suspects disseminated intravascular coagulation (DIC). What imaging feature is most in keeping with pulmonary haemorrhage?
   a Bibasal consolidation and atelectasis
   b Bibasal atelectasis and ground-glass change with small pleural effusions
   c Mid and upper zone patchy consolidation and atelectasis
   d Bilateral patchy segmental and lobar consolidation and ground-glass change
   e Confluent consolidation in a dependent distribution

58 A 62-year-old newspaper editor presented to the Respiratory Clinic with a long history of dyspnoea and daily productive cough. He had smoked 20 cigarettes a day for 45 years. On auscultation there were widespread rhonchi. Pulmonary function tests show a reduced FEV1 and FEV1: FVC ratio, which did not improve with bronchodilator therapy. What are the most likely findings on CT?
   a Varicose bronchial dilatation and lower zone bullous emphysema
   b Centrilobular emphysema in a predominantly mid and upper zone distribution and bronchial wall thickening
   c Panacinar emphysema in a mid and upper zone distribution and cylindrical bronchiole dilatation
   d Lower zone paraseptal emphysema and bronchial wall thickening
   e Mid and lower zone centrilobular emphysema and mild bronchial dilatation

59 A 54-year-old man with a known history of HIV infection presented with a five-day history of severe dyspnoea and malaise but minimal cough. His CD4 count was 90. Bronchoalveolar lavage was performed and a sample showed *Pneumocystis carinii*. What appearance would be likely on his chest radiograph?
   a Unilateral upper zone confluent consolidation and effusion
   b Bilateral lower zone consolidation with small effusions and hilar adenopathy
   c Normal CXR
   d Bilateral perihilar consolidation and ground-glass change
   e Lower-zone bilateral thin-walled cysts

60 The Royal College of Radiologists and the General Medical Council provide guidance on the obtaining of written consent. When is it considered acceptable not to obtain written consent?
   a A complex procedure with significant side-effects
   b A non-therapeutic procedure
   c A procedure where the patient's actions imply consent
   d A procedure that may have consequences on the patient's social life
   e A procedure that is part of a research programme

61 A patient with lower limb ischaemia underwent diagnostic angiography. Therapeutic options including angioplasty, stent insertion, thrombolysis and surgery were considered. When is thrombolysis most appropriate?

a Acute limb ischaemia

b Chronic limb ischaemia

c Claudication

d Irreversible ischaemia

e 'White limb'

62 An 82-year-old arteriopath patient was found to have a palpable pulsatile abdominal mass and ultrasound confirmed an abdominal aortic aneurysm. He was fit enough for either open or endovascular repair and an abdominal CT angiogram was performed to assess suitability for EVAR (endovascular aortic repair). What would make EVAR unfavourable?

a Extension of aneurysm into one common iliac artery

b Infra-renal aneurysm

c Long aneurysmal neck (>15 mm)

d Narrow iliac arteries (<8 mm)

e Neck angulation of 30 degrees

63 An individual underwent a stent graft repair of an infra-renal aneurysm and was followed up with CT aortography the next day. A blush of contrast was seen within the aneurysm sac close to the origin of a small branch from the aorta. What is the next appropriate step in management?

a Prompt surgical correction

b Reduce the systemic blood pressure to less than 120/70

c No immediate intervention: follow up but may be self-limiting

d Reimage only if the patient becomes symptomatic

e Normal finding

64 The right heart border is prominent in a frontal chest radiograph. On the lateral chest radiograph, the anterosuperior aspect of the heart shadow is prominent. Which chamber is likely to be enlarged?

a Right atrium

b Right ventricle

c Left atrium

d Left atrial appendage

e Left ventricle

65 What isolated valve lesion is most likely to cause severe cardiomegaly on a chest radiograph?

a Aortic regurgitation

b Mitral stenosis

c Tricuspid regurgitation

d Pulmonary regurgitation

e Rheumatic heart disease

66 A male infant was born to a mother who had declined all screening during her pregnancy. Labour and delivery were uncomplicated, the infant was of normal birth weight and was well immediately after birth. He then became progressively cyanosed over several hours. What is the most likely underlying diagnosis?
   a Total anomalous pulmonary venous return
   b Transposition of the great vessels
   c Tetralogy of Fallot
   d Pulmonary stenosis
   e Tricuspid atresia

67 A female neonate developed respiratory distress and after investigation was found to have congenital lobar emphysema. Which part of her lung was most likely to have been affected?
   a Right upper lobe
   b Right middle
   c Right lower lobe
   d Left upper lobe
   e Left lower lobe

68 A neonate being treated for necrotising enterocolitis had an umbilical arterial catheter inserted and a check abdominal radiograph was requested. What is the optimal position of the catheter?
   a Passing superiorly from the umbilicus to lie with the tip at the level of the right atrial/IVC junction
   b Passing superiorly from the umbilicus to lie with the tip at T6
   c Passing superiorly from the umbilicus to lie with the tip just inferior to the diaphragm
   d Passing inferiorly from the umbilicus to the pelvis then turning cranially to lie with the tip at T12/L1
   e Passing inferiorly from the umbilicus to the pelvis then turning cranially to lie with the tip at T9

69 A 70-year-old man with chronic obstructive airways disease underwent a CT scan and a tracheal diverticulum was identified. What is the most likely site of this abnormality?
   a Just below the larynx on the left anterolateral wall
   b In the distal trachea on the anterior wall
   c Just above the carina on the posterior wall
   d At the level of the thoracic inlet on the right posterolateral wall
   e At a variable level on the anterior wall

70 A 45-year-old woman with pleuritic chest pain, shortness of breath and profound hypoxia was suspected of having had a pulmonary embolus and a CT pulmonary angiogram was performed. Opacification of the pulmonary vasculature is good with a measured density of 212 HU. What window settings would be optimal when evaluating the pulmonary artery for thrombus?

a Window width 350 HU, window level 40 HU
b Window width 1500 HU, window level –500 HU
c Window width 700 HU, window level 100 HU
d Window width 1500 HU, window level 500 HU
e Window width 100 HU, window level 500 HU

Musculoskeletal and trauma radiology

PAPER 1

1   A young patient, of normal intelligence and with unaffected parents, presented with back pain. The patient was noted to have short limbs and characteristic facial features. Lumbar and thoracic spine plain radiographs showed a decreasing interpedicular distance caudally and posterior scalloping. Which chondroplasia is he most likely to have?
    a   Achondrogenesis
    b   Roberts syndrome
    c   Kniest dysplasia
    d   Achondroplasia
    e   Pseudoachondroplasia

2   A 72-year-old patient on haemodialysis presented with joint pain and effusion of the right shoulder. An arthroscopic specimen stained positive with Congo red. Plain films showed preserved joint space. Which is the most likely diagnosis?
    a   Rheumatoid arthritis
    b   Osteoarthritis
    c   Amyloid arthropathy
    d   Sarcoidosis
    e   Myeloma

3   Which of the following involves avascular necrosis of the vertebral body in patients aged 2–15 years, with normal discs and with an intravertebral vacuum cleft sign?
    a   Legg-Calvé-Perthe disease
    b   Köhler disease
    c   Kienböck's disease
    d   Freiberg disease
    e   Calvé-Kümmel-Verneuil disease

4 An otherwise well 84-year-old woman complains of left knee pain while away on an extended holiday with family and attends a local clinic for analgesia. As part of the work-up a radiograph is performed, which reveals chondro-calcinosis. She also remembers that she has been seen recently by a hospital endocrinologist but cannot remember any further details. What further underlying finding is likely?
a Hypocalcaemia
b Hyperthyroidism
c Hyperparathyroidism
d Hyperkalaemia
e Hypopituitarism

5 A neonate has copious bile-stained vomiting 12 hours after birth. The plain radiograph demonstrates a 'double-bubble' and the paediatrician on call is suspicious that the child has Down syndrome. What bony feature would support this diagnosis?
a Hypotelorism
b A fracture of the odontoid peg
c Avascular necrosis of the femoral head(s)
d Epiphyseal flaring
e Posterior scalloping of the vertebral bodies

6 Of one million people in a region, 100 have ankylosing spondylitis and on average four new cases are diagnosed each year. What is the incidence of ankylosing spondylitis in this population? (Options are cases per million or cases per million per year as appropriate.)
a 4
b 25
c 100
d 104
e 400

7 A bone scan is performed for the investigation of shin splints in a young athlete who complains of lower limb pain on running. Which option best describes the most likely finding in this diagnosis?
a Normal study
b Bilateral symmetrical uptake in the patellae (the 'hot patella sign')
c Linear symmetrical cortical uptake seen most avidly along the posterior aspects of the tibiae
d Linear asymmetrical uptake seen most avidly along the anterior aspects of the tibiae, the 'leading leg' being more avid
e Patchy uptake in the distal tibial shafts

8 A 23-year-old male had a chest radiograph as he was short of breath after falling from his bicycle. The mediastinum and lungs appeared normal but an area of fibrous dysplasia was noted. Which type of fibrous dysplasia is most common?
  a McCune-Albright syndrome
  b Polyostotic
  c Craniofacial
  d Monostotic
  e Familial

9 An 11-year-old girl presented with hip pain and an X-ray of her pelvis was taken. A lucent lesion with an area of periosteal reaction was visible. The periosteal reaction had a 'hair-on-end' configuration. What is the likely nature of any underlying lesion?
  a Normal finding at this age
  b Likely benign tumour
  c Likely aggressive processes
  d Likely haemangioma
  e Non-specific – may be benign or aggressive

10 A 25-year-old man with neurofibromatosis type 1 presents with back pain. What is the most common skeletal abnormality?
  a Widening of intervertebral foramina
  b Anterior scalloping of vertebrae
  c Scoliosis
  d Lordosis
  e Kyphosis

11 A 46-year-old man with haemophilia A has a history of a number of bleeds into the joints of his lower limbs. What feature would be expected on imaging?
  a Uniform sclerosis of all bones
  b A 'squared' patella
  c Expansion of the condylar surface
  d Lateral slanting of tibiotalar joint
  e High signal returned from synovium on T1- and T2-weighted images

12 A seven-year-old child with Marfan syndrome is noted to have an abnormality on a skull X-ray. What is the most likely finding?
  a Osteopenia
  b Dolichocephaly (scaphocephaly)
  c Copper beaten skull
  d Luckenschadel
  e Brachycephaly

13 A 27-year-old patient with poorly developed finger and toe nails presented following a fall onto his knee. An X-ray demonstrated absence of the patella. What further feature would be likely?
a Bilateral posterior iliac horns
b Avascular necrosis of the hip
c Liver dysfunction
d Early onset dementia
e Normal gait

14 You are asked for some advice by a primary care physician who has been consulted by the parents of an 18-month-old child who recently had a series of radiographs of their leg following a fall. No fracture was visible but there is a 1 cm lesion that has been reported as a non-ossifying fibroma. What advice would you convey to the child's parents?
a Need for referral due to risk of pathological fracture
b No need for specific treatment, spontaneous resolution is likely
c Should be treated with high-dose aspirin
d Are associated with Von Hippel-Lindau (VHL) syndrome
e 10% risk of malignant transformation

15 An 80-year-old man presented with right hip pain following a fall was assessed initially with plain radiographs of his hip and pelvis and then a bone scan. What feature would be suggestive of Paget's disease?
a Osseous expansion
b Cortical thinning
c Trabecular thinning
d Thinning of iliopubic and ilioischial lines
e Photopenic lesions on bone scan

16 A 37-year-old man presented as an emergency after falling off his motorbike. He was previously asymptomatic but investigations revealed multiple factures including bilateral femoral fractures and a skull fracture. His bones were noted to be globally abnormal with sclerosis and there was a 'bone within a bone' appearance of several of the vertebrae. Alternating sclerotic and lucent bands were visible in his iliac wings and the base of his skull was noted to be particularly dense. What is the most likely diagnosis?
a Osteomalacia
b Osteopetrosis
c Osteopoikilosis
d Osteoporosis
e Osteosclerosis

17 A 37-year-old female with a long history of right knee pain is eventually diagnosed with pigmented villonodular synovitis (PVNS). What are the most likely findings on imaging?

a Marked joint space narrowing

b High signal of abnormal synovium on all MRI sequences

c Expansion of prefemoral fat pad

d Sclerotic deposits in articular surfaces

e Joint effusion

18 A 46-year-old coal miner with recently diagnosed rheumatoid arthritis was investigated for respiratory symptoms and found to have multiple rapidly developing lung nodules throughout the lungs with a upper and peripheral predominance. What complication is likely to have developed?

a Gaucher's disease

b Caplan's syndrome

c Felty's syndrome

d Acute interstitial pneumonia (AIP)

e Panner's disease

19 A 45-year-old woman with a history of a systemic disease presented with hand pain. What feature would favour a diagnosis of sarcoidosis over scleroderma?

a Reticulated trabecular pattern

b Calcinosis of soft tissues

c Sclerosis of terminal phalanges

d Soft-tissue swelling

e Bony erosions of carpal bones

20 A 56-year-old female patient with stiffness and pain was referred for a radiograph of both hands. What features would favour a diagnosis of psoriatic arthritis over one of rheumatoid arthritis?

a Symmetrical distribution

b Predominant involvement of metacarpophalangeal joints

c Periarticular osteopenia

d Periosteal reaction

e Marginal erosions

21 A 36-year-old man presented with leg pain and an abnormality was noted on the initial radiograph. He then had a bone scan, which appeared normal with no evidence of the abnormality. What would be a possible explanation for this?

a Acute fracture

b Osteomyelitis

c Lymphoma

d Primary hyperparathyroidism

e Paget's disease

22 A 16-year-old athlete presented with a history of locking of his knee following an injury. His plain radiograph demonstrates a small opacity within the joint space. What is the most likely diagnosis?

a Intra-articular loose body
b Calcium pyrophosphate deposition disease (pseudogout)
c Heterotopic ossification
d Anatomical variant
e Osteochondral fracture of the medial femoral condyle

23 A 73-year-old man sustained a ureteric injury during a road traffic accident and is now haemodynamically unstable. What is the most appropriate radiological investigation in the acute setting?

a Contrast-enhanced CT
b Unenhanced CT
c Retrograde urethrography
d One-shot IVU following intravenous contrast medium administration
e Trans-rectal ultrasound (TRUS) of prostate to look for damage to prostatic urethra

24 A series of radiographs of a patient's spine shows hypoplasia of the pedicles, transverse processes and spinous processes. There is also a sharply angled kyphosis in the lower thoracic spine and dural ectasia in the lower lumbar spine with dumbbell-shaped enlargement of a number of the neural foramina. What it the most likely diagnosis?

a Klinefelter's syndrome
b Neurofibromatosis type 1
c Down syndrome
d Tuberous sclerosis
e Von Hippel-Lindau syndrome

25 A 20-year old man jumped 30 feet from a building onto concrete and landed on his feet. He was assessed in the Emergency Department and complained only of severe pain in his feel. He remained haemodynamically stable and after a full assessment it is clear that his only injuries are to his feet. What injury is he most likely to have sustained?

a Osteochondral fracture of talar dome
b March fractures of second and third metatarsals
c Comminuted calcaneal fractures
d Maisonneuve fracture
e Transverse fracture of fifth metatarsal

26 A 46-year-old woman is brought into the emergency room after a road traffic accident. She was the driver and had a high-speed collision with a parked van. She responds to pain and is haemodynamically stable. There are no obvious bony or visceral injuries on either primary or secondary survey. She has had an urgent CT head, which revealed no abnormality and her C-spine is clear. As the on-call radiologist you are asked to review her chest X-ray, which shows a widened mediastinum. There are no previous studies available for comparison. What should the subsequent radiological management be?

  a Transthoracic echocardiography
  b Cardiac MRI
  c Lateral chest X-ray
  d Contrast-enhanced CT chest
  e No imaging, transfer directly to theatre for thoracotomy

27 An elderly lady fell onto her back and experienced severe back and buttock pain. Pelvic radiographs revealed marked osteopenia but no definite fracture. A bone scan was then performed, which showed an H-shaped pattern of increased uptake. Which bone is likely to be involved?

  a Sacrum
  b Ilium
  c Ischium
  d Pubis
  e Fifth lumbar vertebra

28 A woman with poorly controlled diabetes mellitus fell down the stairs feet first. She did not experience much pain but found it difficult to walk after the fall and visited the Emergency Department where a doctor noticed that her ankle joint appeared abnormal with a large haematoma on the medial aspect of her foot. Neurological examination demonstrated bilateral sensory impairment in a stocking distribution. What injury is she most likely to have sustained?

  a Osteochondral fracture of the talar dome
  b Fracture of the medial malleolus
  c Maisonneuve fracture
  d Lisfranc fracture-dislocation
  e Pilon fracture

29 A 44-year-old man had an accident in which he was thrown from a motorcycle. He landed on his left foot, which folded beneath him. On the day of the injury, his foot was examined and standard AP and lateral radiographs revealed no fracture. The foot was placed in slight plantar flexion and immobilised with a cast. After three days, the patient was re-evaluated and his foot remained oedematous. Ecchymoses was noted laterally and he could not weight-bear. What injury is he most likely to have sustained?

  a No bony or ligamentous injury is likely
  b Torn ligament between the second metatarsal and medial cuneiform

   c Transverse fracture through base of fifth metatarsal

   d Fracture of second metacarpal associated with dislocation of the tarsometatarsal joint

   e Fracture of medial malleolus

30 A 56-year-old plumber complained of long-standing bilateral pain anterior to his knees. There was no history of trauma although he reports spending two hours a day kneeling. AP, lateral and skyline radiographs of both knees showed soft-tissue swelling anterior to the patella but no bony abnormality. What is the most appropriate further management?

   a 1.5T MRI

   b Unenhanced CT

   c 3.0T MRI

   d Arthroscopy

   e No further imaging – rest and occupational modification alone are adequate

31 A 26-year-old woman suffered an assault in which she sustained a blow to the right side of her chin. She was unable to close her mouth fully and her incisors were chipped. An orthopantomograph (OPG) examination revealed a mandibular fracture. At what anatomical site is the fracture most likely?

   a Mandibular condyle

   b Ramus of mandible

   c Coronoid process of mandible

   d Parasymphyseal

   e Body of mandible

32 A 94-year-old lady was found on the floor in her nursing home. On arrival to the Emergency Department the attending doctor noticed a shortened and externally rotated right leg and radiographs of the right hip were requested. These show a minimally displaced fracture just below the right femoral neck and just above the greater and lesser trochanters. What is the treatment of choice?

   a Dynamic hip screw

   b Uncemented hemi-arthroplasty

   c Cannulated screws

   d Femoral head resurfacing

   e Total hip replacement

33 A football goalkeeper dived to the ground while making a save and experienced immediate pain in his wrist. The action replay shows forced hyperextension in ulnar deviation. Radiographs reveal no abnormality on the AP projection, but a subtle fracture on the lateral view. What bone is most likely to have been injured?
a Capitate
b Hamate
c Lunate
d Pisiform
e Triquetral

34 A skier fell on his outstretched hand with his hand caught in his ski pole and sustained an abduction injury of his thumb. His thumb was painful and swollen and he noticed that it felt unstable. He consulted a doctor in the resort who arranged radiographs of his hand and wrist. What is the most likely diagnosis?
a Dislocation of carpo-metacarpal joint of thumb
b Soft-tissue injury only
c Scaphoid fracture
d Rupture of ulnar collateral ligament
e Dislocation of first metacarpophalangeal joint

35 A 47-year-old woman sustained a significant flexion injury to the cervical spine as a result of a high-velocity road traffic accident. Her spine was immobilised and she was taken to the local trauma centre for assessment. A lateral cervical spine radiograph revealed 50% anterolisthesis of C4 on C5 and malalignment of the apophyseal joints. There was no suggestion of a rotational component to the injury. What type of injury is this?
a Stable unilateral facet dislocation
b Unstable unilateral facet dislocation
c Bilateral facet dislocation
d Jefferson fracture
e Perched facets

36 A 17-year-old male was found to have a 3-cm lytic lesion surrounded by marked sclerosis in the distal diaphysis of his right femur. CT confirmed the presence of a nidus with matrix mineralisation and there was no suspicion of other lesions. What is the most likely diagnosis?
a Osteoblastoma
b Enchondroma
c Giant cell tumour
d Ewing sarcoma
e Fibrous dysplasia

37 A middle-aged gentleman who is otherwise well was shown to have coarse, vertically aligned trabeculae on a lumbar spine radiograph. A comprehensive

range of blood tests were all normal. A CT of his spine was performed which showed a 'pepperpot' pattern with small dots of high density on axial images. The cortical margins were well preserved. What is the most likely diagnosis?

a Paget's disease

b Haemangioma

c Metastatic prostate carcinoma

d Multiple myeloma

e Lymphoma

38 Which childhood tumour is almost exclusively located in the epiphysis?

a Osteosarcoma

b Lymphoma

c Chondroblastoma

d Ewing sarcoma

e Non-ossifying fibroma

39 You are preparing the equipment required to perform a bone biopsy. When would a coaxial (introducer-sheathed) needle offer an advantage?

a To biopsy a deep lesion

b To biopsy a superficial lesion

c To biopsy a large, easy to target lesion

d To obtain a larger specimen

e To reduce cost

40 A 40-year-old man presented with lethargy and knee pain. A radiograph showed a diaphyseal lesion with bone destruction. What diagnosis would be most likely?

a Osteoblastoma

b Non-ossifying fibroma

c Lymphoma

d Chondroblastoma

e Aneurysmal bone cyst

41 A 67-year-old man was noticed to have a mixed sclerotic and lucent region in his proximal tibia with bowing of the bone and marked thickening of the cortex. There was no periosteal reaction. What is the most likely diagnosis?

a Paget's disease

b Aneurysmal bone cyst

c Rickets

d Non-ossifying fibroma

e Chondromyxoid fibroma

42 A 35-year-old lady with a two-month history of pain, localised swelling and reduced range of movement of her right knee was shown to have a lytic subarticular lesion in the epiphysis and metaphysis of her distal femur. No surrounding sclerosis or soft-tissue swelling was seen. A subsequent MRI showed heterogeneous signal on both T1- and T2-weighted images. No fluid/fluid levels were visible. What is the most likely diagnosis?

a Metastatic breast deposit
b Enchondroma
c Aneurysmal bone cyst
d Desmoplastic fibroma
e Giant cell tumour

43 A 38-year-old female presented with a large, destructive giant cell tumour in her distal femur. What is the most appropriate management?

a Wide resection and reconstruction with allograft
b Curettage and bone graft
c Embolisation
d Radiotherapy
e Conservative management
f Chemotherapy

44 A 22-year-old man presented with pain and swelling of his right knee having knocked it while playing football. The X-ray revealed a destructive lesion in the proximal tibia with a mixed sclerotic/lytic appearance. A 'hair on end' type periosteal reaction was also visible. An MRI showed intermediate signal with foci of high signal intensity on T1- and heterogeneous high-signal T2-weighted images. What is the most likely diagnosis?

a Osteoid osteoma
b Osteochondroma
c Osteosarcoma
d Chondromyxoid fibroma
e Chondrosarcoma

45 A 19-year-old girl presented with discomfort in her left leg of gradual onset with no history of trauma. A radiograph showed a translucent area with a thin sclerotic rim in the epiphysis of her left femur. An MRI was subsequently performed to further characterise this lesion and showed a lobulated margin of low signal intensity corresponding to the sclerotic margin on the X-ray. What is the most likely diagnosis?

a Clear cell chondrosarcoma
b Chondroblastoma
c Osteosarcoma
d Fibrosarcoma
e Osteoma

45 A 20-year-old man slowly developed predominantly nocturnal low back pain. He reports that salicylate-based medication is particularly helpful in relieving his pain. What is the most likely diagnosis?

a Fibrosarcoma

b Malignant fibrous histiocytoma

c Osteoid osteoma

d Chondrosarcoma

e Ollier's disease

46 A 76-year-old man presented with pain in his left femur. There was a long history of Paget's disease and bony tenderness about his knee on the medial femoral condyle. He denied any history of trauma and a radiograph showed an area with sunburst periosteal reaction within the Pagetoid bone. What is the most likely diagnosis?

a Osteosarcoma

b Osteochondroma

c Chondrosarcoma

d Fibrous dysplasia

e Osteomalacia

47 A 12 year old was shown to have an eccentric, lobulated lesion involving the cortex and medulla of the proximal tibial metaphysis with a sclerotic endosteal border but no periosteal reaction. A subsequent CT showed no soft-tissue extension or fluid levels. What is the most likely diagnosis?

a Aneurysmal bone cyst

b Enchondroma

c Chondrosarcoma

d Polyostotic fibrous dysplasia

e Chondromyxoid fibroma

48 An 11-year-old boy with hip pain was found to have an osteoid osteoma of his right neck of femur. What is the most appropriate treatment of this lesion?

a Chemotherapy

b Resection and prosthetic replacement

c Percutaneous radiofrequency ablation (RFA)

d Low-dose focal irradiation (800 cGy)

e Curettage, cryotherapy and bone grafting

49 A patient presented with a long history of pain in her wrist and no history of trauma. A radiograph showed a sharply marginated lesion with multiple foci of 'popcorn'-like calcification. Bone densitometry was within normal limits. An MRI showed hypointensity to muscle on both T1- and T2-weighted images and no fluid collections. What is the most likely diagnosis?

a Fibrous dysplasia

b Osteogenesis imperfecta

c Multiple enchondromas

d Calcifying solitary bone cyst

e Aneurysmal bone cyst

50 A 27-year-old Afro-Caribbean patient with known sickle cell disease presented with ongoing pain left arm pain following a crisis and was found to have osteomyelitis of his humerus. What is the most likely causative organism?

a *Proteus mirabilis*

b *Escherichia coli*

c *Staphylococcus aureus*

d *Mycoplasma pneumoniae*

e *Corynebacterium diphtheriae*

51 A mildly expansile lytic lesion was noted in the femur of an otherwise well 14-year-old boy. This was well defined and unilocular and extended from metaphysis into diaphysis. The remaining bone was well mineralised and there were no associated aggressive features. What is the most likely diagnosis?

a Aneurysmal bone cyst

b Fibrous dysplasia

c Giant cell tumour

d Simple bone cyst

e Brown tumour

52 A six-year-old child presented unwell with a history of 12 weeks of pain and swelling over the left knee. On examination they were pyrexial and noted to have a knee effusion. Blood tests showed a raised erythrocyte sedimentation rate (ESR) and a radiograph showed an aggressive destructive lesion with a permeative pattern of bone destruction in the distal femur and a lamellated ('onion skin') periosteal reaction. What is the most likely diagnosis?

a Ewing sarcoma

b Brodie's abscess

c Trauma

d Secondary neuroblastoma

e Eosinophilic granuloma

53 A 15-year-old boy was recently diagnosed with a Ewing sarcoma of his vertebral column. Which segment is most likely to be affected?
   a Cervical spine
   b Thoracic spine
   c Lumbar spine
   d Sacrum
   e Coccyx

54 A six-year-old boy was brought to the GP with his parents after sudden onset of pain in the proximal humerus. Radiographs reveal fracture through a simple bone cyst. What imaging features would be most typical?
   a Thick internal septa
   b Well-defined lucency but no sclerotic rim
   c Subarticular epiphyseal location
   d Long axis perpendicular to bone
   e Thinned cortex with mild expansion

55 A 32-year-old man presents with pain and swelling in his right shoulder of four years' duration that has gradually been getting worse recently. He works as a mechanic and has been having increasing difficulty using his right arm for the last few months but is otherwise well. On examination he has an obviously swollen right shoulder. A firm mass is palpable over the lateral aspect of his proximal humerus, extending distally to his elbow. There are also multiple palpable axillary lymph nodes. A radiograph of his shoulder shows a mottled, permeative lucency in the head of the humerus. What is the most likely diagnosis?
   a Eosinophilic granuloma
   b Ewing sarcoma
   c Metastatic deposit
   d Non-Hodgkin's lymphoma
   e Osteomyelitis

56 A nine-year-old girl presented with pain and swelling of her left lower leg over the anteromedial aspect of her tibia. A radiograph showed an aggressive lesion with mixed lytic/sclerotic appearances in the proximal tibial metaphysis. A biopsy was taken which showed odd-looking pleomorphic cells and stained positive for osteoid. What is the most likely diagnosis?
   a Granulocytic sarcoma
   b Ewing sarcoma
   c Osteosarcoma
   d Aneurysmal bone cyst
   e Osteoid osteoma

57 A five-year-old boy was noted to have multiple hard swellings predominately around his knees, and radiographs showed multiple bony outgrowths extending laterally from the bone and pointing away from the nearest joint. The overlying cortex remained in continuity with the native bone although there were some modelling deformities associated with the lesions. What are the individual lesions?

   a Osteosarcoma
   b Osteochondroma
   c Chondroblastoma
   d Chondrosarcoma
   e Ivory osteoma

58 A 16-year-old female was investigated for a lucent lesion in her spine and a primary bone tumour was suspected. As part of the work-up a three-phase bone scan was performed and the lesion of interest showed high activity in the blood-pool phase. What is the most likely diagnosis?

   a Chondroma
   b Simple bone cyst
   c Aneurysmal bone cyst
   d Chondromyxoid fibroma
   e Enostosis (bone island)

59 A 25-year-old patient presented with back pain and was found to have a single abnormally dense vertebra, which remained of normal size and shape. The endplates were of normal appearance. What diagnosis is the most likely?

   a Haemangioma
   b Ankylosing spondylitis
   c Metastatic deposit from thyroid carcinoma
   d Osteomyelitis
   e Sclerotic osteosarcoma

60 A 39-year-old male presented with a long history of back pain and was eventually diagnosed with an ependymoma. Where was this lesion most likely to have occurred?

   a Within the skull
   b Cervical spine
   c Thoracic spine
   d Lumbar spine
   e Sacrum

61 Which statement best describes the characteristics of a chondromyxoid fibroma?

   a Geographic bone destruction with periosteal reaction
   b Poorly defined lesion with no sclerotic rim and septation
   c Geographic bone destruction with no sclerotic rim

    d Poorly defined lucency with periosteal reaction and expansions

    e Geographic bone destruction with a prominent sclerotic rim

62 At what age does a chondroblastoma usually present?
    a 0–5 years
    b 10–20 years
    c 30–40 years
    d 50–60 years
    e Over 70 years

63 How are enchondromas most likely to present?
    a Anaemia
    b Fever
    c Malaise
    d Malignant degeneration
    e Pathologic fracture

64 A 42-year-old patient was investigated for acute abdominal pain and had a CT. There were features of inflammatory bowel disease and an incidental finding of a haemangioma in the L1 vertebra. Which part of the vertebra is most likely to be involved?
    a Spinous process
    b Pars articularis
    c Transverse process
    d Pedicles
    e Vertebral body

65 What is the sex distribution of patients who develop Ewing sarcoma?
    a 4 Male: 1 Female
    b 2 Male: 1 Female
    c 1 Male: 1 Female
    d 1 Male: 2 Female
    e 1 Male: 4 Female

66 A 40-year-old female presented feeling unwell and was found to have a raised serum calcium and alkaline phosphatase with a borderline low phosphate. She had several recent episodes of renal colic and felt generally weak. An X-ray of her pelvis showed a lytic lesion that was associated with an underlying endocrine abnormality. What is the likely imaging appearance?
    a Poorly defined central lesion with prominent periosteal reaction
    b Poorly defined eccentric lesion with periosteal reaction
    c Poorly defined central lesion with no periosteal reaction
    d Well-defined cortical lesion with no periosteal reaction
    e Well-defined central lesion with prominent periosteal reaction

67 A young adult female with severe acne had several episodes of inflammatory joint symptoms and a radiograph of her knee showed juxtaarticular osteoporosis. She also had evidence of osteosclerosis of several vertebrae with paravertebral ossification. What other skin rash is she at high risk of?
a Erythema nodosum
b Heliotrope rash
c Palmoplantar pustulosis
d Pemphigus
e Psoriasis

68 A five-year-old boy injured his leg in the playground and a radiograph was obtained the same day. This demonstrated a pseudoarthrosis of the fibula. What is the most likely underlying diagnosis?
a Non-union of fracture
b Osteomyelitis
c Neurofibromatosis
d Chondroectodermal dysplasia (Ellis-van Creveld syndrome)
e Holt-Oram syndrome

69 A patient presented with pneumonia and had a chest radiograph. This showed absence of the clavicles, 13 pairs of ribs and a narrowed thorax. What is the likely inheritance of the underlying condition?
a X-linked
b Spontaneous mutation
c Mitochondrial
d Autosomal recessive
e Autosomal dominant

70 A 30-year-old man had a shoulder radiograph following an injury that showed no fracture, but there were multiple small (up to 6 mm) ovoid bone islands throughout the bones with the long axis running parallel to the bone. He remembered that his father had a similar condition and asks whether it puts him at an increased risk of malignancy. What is the increased risk?
a No increased risk
b High risk of colorectal carcinoma
c High risk of osteosarcoma
d Moderate increased risk of colorectal carcinoma
e Moderate increased risk of osteosarcoma

Musculoskeletal and trauma radiology

PAPER 2

1   A 40-year-old female presents with a three-month history of headaches and a visual field defect. An MRI of the sella turcica diagnosed a growth hormone-secreting pituitary adenoma. Which of the following findings would you expect on plain radiography?
    a   Heel pad thickness >25 mm
    b   Opacification of paranasal sinuses
    c   Thinned skull vault
    d   Reduction in size of vertebral bodies
    e   Increased cortical thickness of long bones

2   A 17-year-old female presented with foot pain on walking. Plain films showed a well-defined cystic lesion in the second metatarsal head. What is a plain film six months later likely to show?
    a   Cortical thinning
    b   Sclerosis and flattening of the second metatarsal head
    c   Sclerosis of the other metatarsals
    d   Subluxation of the metatarsal heads
    e   Bony erosions in the metatarsal heads

3   A fit and well 72-year-old female presented to her general practitioner with medial knee pain, having twisted her knee four months previously. Initial films on attendance at the Emergency Department at the time of the injury were reported as normal. Repeat films several months later on showed flattening of part of the medial condyle and a radiolucent focus. Which of the following is the most likely diagnosis?
    a   Panner's disease
    b   Metastasis
    c   Benign cortical defect
    d   Lymphoma
    e   Spontaneous osteonecrosis of the knee

4 A 42-year-old secretary complains of pain and tingling in the radial three and one-half digits of the palmar surface of her right hand. Her symptoms began almost a year ago with nocturnal burning and tingling and have progressed since then. Her thenar eminence shows early wasting. An MRI of her wrist is arranged for further assessment. What features would be expected?

a Increased signal intensity of the median nerve on T2WI
b Decreased signal of the median nerve on T1WI
c Dorsal bowing of flexor retinaculum
d Normal nerve diameter inside the carpal tunnel
e Thickening of the ligament of Struthers

5 A 17-year-old patient with Ehlers-Danlos syndrome is due for further investigations. What investigation would be contraindicated?

a Aortography
b Barium enema
c Intravenous urogram
d CT brain
e Tc-99m bone scan

6 A 69-year-old female who had a right total knee replacement four years ago returns to clinic with knee pain. Her inflammatory markers and plain films are normal. A three-phase bone scan shows no increased uptake on dynamic or blood pool images, but static images show focal linear horizontal uptake in the medial tibial compartment adjacent to tibial component. Which is the most likely explanation?

a Early loosening of prosthesis
b Subclinical infection
c Weight-bearing load area of knee producing uptake
d Normal findings at this post-operative stage
e Referred pain from hip

7 A 62-year-old patient with non-specific bone pain is referred for a bone scan, which shows avid diffuse uptake in the right femur corresponding to a thickened cortical outline. The bone scan is otherwise normal for age. What is the most likely diagnosis?

a Monostotic fibrous dysplasia
b Monostotic Paget's disease
c Osteomalacia and insufficiency fracture
d Myelofibrosis
e Osteosarcoma

8 A 38-year-old man presented with a lump on the dorsal aspect of his hand that moved with the tendons on flexion and extension of his fingers. An X-ray and then MRI of this area were performed. What imaging findings might be expected?

a A dense calcified mass
b Low signal on T2-weighted images
c High signal on T1-weighted images
d No internal septations
e Periosteal new bone formation

9 A 10-year-old schoolboy had a fall and bruised his right knee badly. There was an open wound that was not treated until the following day. After a further two days he became systemically unwell with a fever. His knee was extremely tender, swollen, and the movement was restricted. Which of the following is a feature of septic arthritis?
a Usually due to *Haemophilus*
b Periarticular soft tissue swelling is rare
c Blurring of the periarticular fat planes is common
d The joint space widens after a few weeks
e A joint effusion is not usually present

10 A 50-year-old man is known to have haemochromatosis and presents with pain in his hands. What distribution of involvement would be typical?
a Interphalangeal joint of thumb
b Proximal interphalangeal joints of all fingers
c Distal interphalangeal joints of middle and ring fingers
d Metacarpophalangeal joints of index and middle fingers
e Metacarpophalangeal joints of ring and little fingers

11 A 55 year old with a history of several severe attacks of rheumatic fever presented with a polyarthropathy affecting the metacarpophalangeal joints of both hands with ulnar deviation and subluxation. The joint spaces were preserved and they were able to voluntarily correct the subluxation. What is the most likely diagnosis?
a Jaccoud's arthropathy
b Rheumatoid arthropathy
c Amyloid arthropathy
d Psoriatic arthritis
e Haemophilic arthropathy

12 A 17-year-old boy presented to the Emergency Department five weeks after falling off his bike and hitting his thigh. Plain films showed some faint calcifications in the tissue adjacent to the femur and some simple periosteal reaction. A CT scan confirmed peripheral ossification. What is the most likely diagnosis?
a Osteosarcoma
b Fibrosarcoma
c Stress fracture
d Chondrosarcoma
e Myositis ossificans

13 A 56-year-old woman presented with an ankle deformity and was found to have reduced proprioception of this leg such that it was only minimally tender despite dislocation and marked bone destruction being visible on radiographs. What is a possible underlying cause?

a Charcot-Marie-Tooth

b Hyperthyroidism

c Prolonged use of antibiotics

d Acromegaly

e Use of hyoscine butylbromide (Buscopan®)

14 A 38-year-old female with a history of iron deficiency anaemia is seen in the Emergency Department following an alleged assault and has a skull radiograph to exclude the presence of a foreign body. What feature would be suggestive of a recurrence of her anaemia?

a Narrowing of diploe

b Hair-on-end appearance of skull

c Osteopenia of zygoma

d Osteosclerosis of sphenoid

e Biconcave vertebrae

15 An elderly woman with known Paget's disease of her skull presented following a fall. According to her husband she had also been becoming more confused recently. What feature secondary to Paget's disease is most likely?

a Osteoblastoma

b Cerebral hemisphere compression

c Hydrocephalus

d Hypocalcaemia

e Leukaemia

16 A 67-year-old woman with known rheumatoid arthritis presented with right shoulder pain and a radiograph was performed. There was no history of trauma and secondary osteoarthritis was not thought to be a dominant feature. What features would be typical?

a Subchondral lucency

b Osteophytosis of the glenoid

c Increased joint space

d Widened glenohumeral joint space

e Tapered margin of distal clavicle

17 An overweight 12-year-old boy was noticed to be limping at school. There is no history of trauma but he remembers some stiffness in the right hip over the last few weeks, which improved with rest. A radiograph of the pelvis shows that a line drawn along the superior edge of the femoral neck (Klein's line) does not intersect the femoral head. What is the most likely diagnosis?

a Septic arthritis

b Perthes' disease

c Developmental dysplasia of the hip (DDH)

d Slipped upper femoral epiphysis (SUFE)

e Blount's disease

18 A 50-year-old man presented with foot pain and radiographs showed involvement of a number of joints with generally non-specific findings. What underlying diagnosis would the presence of periostitis favour?

a Gout

b Pseudogout

c Psoriatic arthritis

d Haemophilia

e Rheumatoid arthritis

19 A 19-year-old woman was investigated for foot stiffness and was found to have a tarsal coalition. What type of coalition is she most likely to have?

a Calcaneocuboid

b Calcaneonavicular

c Cubonavicular

d Cuneometatarsal

e Talonavicular

20 A patient with a chromosomal disorder was noted to have a number of musculoskeletal abnormalities. What feature would favour the diagnosis of Turner's syndrome over Down syndrome?

a Atlantoaxial subluxation

b Tall stature

c Madelung's deformity

d Gracile ribs

e Anterior scalloping of vertebral bodies

21 A 60-year-old woman with a history of breast cancer 10 years previously presented with back pain and a bone scan was arranged. Other than metastatic disease, what would be a cause of increased uptake?

a Multiple myeloma

b Dental disease

c Haemangioma

d Acute fracture

e Radiotherapy field

22 A 22-year-old man who was an unrestrained back-seat passenger was involved in a high-speed road traffic accident and sustained an aortic injury. Which part of his aorta is most likely to have been injured?
   a Aortic root
   b Ascending aorta just before origin of brachiocephalic artery
   c Between brachiocephalic and left common carotid arteries
   d Just distal to left subclavian artery
   e Aortic hiatus (level of diaphragm)

23 A 25-year-old motorcyclist who was in collision with a bus is being treated for a pelvic fracture and haematuria. On examination he has perineal ecchymoses. He is due to have a CT for further assessment of his urinary tract. How long after injection of 100 mL of low osmolar iodinated contrast at 3.5 mL/second into the antecubital fossa should images be acquired?
   a Immediately
   b 25 seconds
   c 60 seconds
   d 4 minutes
   e 30 minutes

24 A 12-year-old boy presented with a painful, swollen left knee after a football injury. AP and lateral radiographs of the knee demonstrated a bone fragment on the lateral aspect of the knee that was felt to be secondary to popliteus tendon avulsion. What is the function of the popliteus muscle?
   a It locks the knee
   b It is an extensor of the knee joint
   c It controls lateral meniscal displacement
   d It limits anterior tibial translation
   e It is a flexor of the knee joint

25 A young girl dived into a shallow swimming pool and struck the bottom of the pool head first. She was brought to the Emergency Department where she was drowsy and on examination there was a large scalp haematoma and some upper cervical spine tenderness. Which of the following would be the most appropriate imaging?
   a CT head and lateral C-spine radiograph
   b Skull radiograph and MRI of neck
   c CT head and AP C-spine radiograph
   d Skull, AP and lateral C-spine radiographs
   e CT head and cervical spine

26 A 17-year-old teenager was involved in a fight and presented to the Emergency Department with a severely bruised and swollen hand. What fracture is he most likely to have sustained?
a Fracture of the shaft of the fifth metacarpal
b Intra-articular fracture of the base of the first metacarpal
c Fracture of the scaphoid waist
d Rolando fracture
e Triquetral fracture

27 A 55-year-old lady with rheumatoid arthritis presented to the Emergency Department with sudden onset pain and swelling on the medial side of her left foot. Clinical examination revealed marked weakness of plantar flexion and inversion on the left, but normal power on the right. What tendon is most likely to have been injured?
a Extensor digitorum
b Peroneus tertius
c Tibialis anterior
d Flexor hallucis longus
e Tibialis posterior

28 A 15-year-old schoolboy suffered an assault with a baseball bat. He was taken by ambulance to the Emergency Department where he was initially fully conscious but subsequently became comatose. After assessment with CT, a neurosurgical intervention produced an excellent recovery. What is the most likely appearance on the CT?
a Small high-attenuation foci throughout the cerebral cortices
b Hydrocephalus
c A bi-convex collection of high density adjacent to a linear lucency in the skull vault
d A crescentic extra-axial collection of mixed attenuation
e A low attenuation collection in the right occipital region with an area of high attenuation in the left frontal region

29 A 64-year-old man was involved in a high-speed road traffic accident. He had been wearing a seatbelt and there was no evidence of external injury, but he arrived at the local Trauma Centre in haemodynamic shock. His abdomen became tense and distended and there was a profound acidosis on arterial blood gas analysis. A CT scan was performed and a bowel/mesenteric injury was suspected. What findings on CT are most sensitive for surgically important bowel or mesenteric injury?
a Mesenteric vessel extravasation
b Mesenteric air
c Intraperitoneal free fluid
d Abnormal bowel wall enhancement
e Focal mesenteric haematoma

30 A 44-year-old taxi driver was involved in a 40-mph collision with a stationary car. After assessment he was found to have a stable fracture of his cervical spine and was discharged from hospital. What injury is he most likely to have sustained?

   a Posterior arch fracture of the atlas
   b Flexion teardrop fracture
   c Chance fracture
   d Clay-shoveller's fracture
   e Bilateral interfacetal dislocation of C3/4

31 A footballer was tackled from behind while playing in his local park. He felt a sudden 'pop' and his knee became swollen and unstable. While waiting for an MRI scan he noticed his leg pivoted outward about his knee as he walked. What are the most likely findings on the MRI scan?

   a MCL rupture due to valgus stress
   b LCL rupture due to direct blow
   c MCL rupture due to varus stress
   d LCL rupture due to varus stress
   e MCL rupture due direct blow

32 A 54-year old lady presented with severe progressive pain in her lumbar spine. As she had a past history of breast cancer (treated with a wide local excision and radiotherapy) a Technetium-99 bone scan was requested. This showed diffuse uptake throughout the lumbar vertebrae and ribs. Which of the following anatomical sites is most suggestive of metastatic bony disease?

   a Vertebral body
   b Lamina
   c Pedicle
   d Sternum
   e Superior articular facet

33 A 35-year-old horse rider complains of severe pain in her left thigh after riding a horse for the first time in many weeks. She has recently returned from a long business trip where she was unable to do any horse riding or other physical activity while away. The clinical team request an ultrasound scan to confirm the clinical diagnosis. What is the most likely abnormality?

   a Focus of low echogenicity within quadriceps tendon
   b Discontinuity of sartorius tendon
   c High echogenicity foci within gluteus maximus muscle belly
   d Low attenuation within biceps femoris muscle belly
   e Discontinuity of musculotendinous junction of adductor longus muscle

34 A 17-year-old girl attempted suicide by jumping from the second floor of her apartment building. She landed such that her left leg sustained almost all the impact of her fall. When seen in the Emergency Department she was fully alert, having sustained no head, chest, spinal or abdominal injuries. Her left leg was severely bruised with an open wound and the right leg and foot appeared normal. Radiographs revealed a comminuted distal tibial fracture with intra-articular involvement associated with a fracture of the mid-shaft of the left fibula. What type of injury is this?

a Maisonneuve fracture
b Torus fracture
c Osteochondral fracture
d Pilon fracture
e Lisfranc fracture

35 A 25-year-old man suffered a severe blow to the side of his face during an assault. He was unable to open his mouth and severe bruising with flattening of the contour of his cheek was visible on initial presentation to hospital. Facial radiographs were performed and a facial fracture was visible that was most clearly seen on the submentovertex view. What is the most likely diagnosis?

a Zygomatic arch fracture
b Le Fort I fracture
c Le Fort III fracture
d Coronoid process fracture
e Orbital blowout fracture

36 A 17-year-old female noticed pain and swelling around her distal thigh, particularly while exercising. She had no history of trauma. On examination there was localised tenderness above her knee. Radiographically, a lytic expansile lesion in the metaphysis of the distal femur surrounded by a very thin rim of cortex was visible. There was no periosteal reaction. What is the most likely disease process?

a Ewing sarcoma
b Osteosarcoma
c Fibrous dysplasia
d Aneurysmal bone cyst
e Chondrosarcoma

37 A 14-year-old boy with a three-week history of persistent pain in his right leg presented to hospital. He was noted to have a temperature of 37.8°C and a radiograph of his leg showed a diaphyseal mass in the right femur with overlying cortical erosion and soft-tissue swelling. A bone biopsy was undertaken showing numerous small round blue cells. Which of the following tumours is he most likely to have?
a Neuroblastoma
b Medulloblastoma metastasis
c Osteoblastoma
d Ewing's sarcoma
e Chondroblastoma

38 A 12 year old presented with a large lesion in their distal femur. What approach would be most appropriate for bone biopsy?
a Medial approach
b Lateral approach
c Posterior approach
d Anterior approach
e Trans-venous percutaneous approach

39 An elderly gentleman presented with a two-month history of back pain. There was no history of significant osteoarthritis and no history of trauma. Plain radiographs revealed multiple sclerotic lesions scattered throughout the spine, which were confirmed as sites of increased uptake on a Tc-99 radionuclide bone scan. What primary tumour is most likely?
a Breast
b Thyroid
c Kidney
d Prostate
e Lung

40 A 21-year-old man presented with pain in his knee following a fall and a radiograph demonstrated a bone tumour in his patella. What lesion is most likely?
a Osteosarcoma
b Osteochondroma
c Chondroblastoma
d Non-ossifying fibroma
e Adamantinoma

41 A 14-year-old female presented with arm pain with no history of trauma and was found to have an eccentric non-expansile lucent lesion in her proximal humerus. There was no soft tissue mass or periosteal reaction and a subsequent MRI showed multiple fluid-fluid levels. What is the most likely diagnosis?
   a Giant cell tumour
   b Aneurysmal bone cyst
   c Enchondroma
   d Osteoblastoma
   e Fibrous dysplasia

42 A 26-year-old woman was found to have a suspected giant cell tumour in her proximal humerus. What is the most appropriate management?
   a Biopsy and surgical curettage, no follow-up required
   b Biopsy, 'extended' curettage and packing with follow-up X-rays
   c Curettage alone
   d Biopsy with follow up X-rays
   e Conservative management

43 A 30-year-old man was found to have monostotic fibrous dysplasia affecting his humerus. Which part of the bone is more likely to be involved?
   a Epiphyseal
   b Epiphyseal and metaphyseal
   c Metaphyseal
   d Metaphyseal and diaphyseal
   e Diaphyseal

44 A 22-year-old man was found to have an osteosarcoma of his proximal tibia. How should this patient be managed?
   a Curettage and bone grafting
   b Above knee amputation
   c Wide resection only
   d Wide resection and chemotherapy
   e Wide resection and radiotherapy

45 A 55-year-old man presented with leg pain and a suspicious lesion was seen on a radiograph. Bone biopsy showed an osteogenic sarcoma and referral to the regional oncology centre was undertaken. What is the most important initial staging investigation?
   a Chest X-ray
   b MRI brain
   c Lymphoscintigram
   d US liver
   e IVU renal tract

46 A 68-year-old man presents with insidious onset right-sided shoulder pain. He gives no history of trauma but has recently lost some weight. On examination, he has a markedly reduced range of movement of the shoulder with a palpable mass. An AP radiograph shows 'popcorn' calcification in the head of the humerus. What is the most likely diagnosis?
   a Chondroblastoma
   b Osteosarcoma
   c Chondrosarcoma
   d Multiple myeloma
   e Desmoplastic fibroma

47 A 27-year-old female with a long-standing history of back pain was found to have a scoliosis. A plain radiograph demonstrated the absence of the right pedicle of T9 and a bone scan showed a hot spot at this site. CT confirmed a lytic expansile lesion with an associated soft-tissue mass. Biopsy showed the lesion to be benign and as the patient declined treatment, follow-up showed slow growth. What is the most likely diagnosis?
   a Aneurysmal bone cyst
   b Osteoblastoma
   c Osteoid osteoma
   d Chondromyxoid fibroma
   e Langerhans cell histiocytosis

48 A 12-year-old boy presented with pain in his thigh for a period of three weeks, which is worse at night and relieved by aspirin. Radiographs showed a small lucent area in the proximal femoral cortex surrounded by sclerosis. What is the most likely diagnosis?
   a Osteochondroma
   b Eosinophilic granuloma
   c Multiple myeloma
   d Enchondroma
   e Osteoid osteoma

49 A nine-year-old girl with past history of cyclical vaginal bleeding presented with an eight-month history of hip and ankle pain. Multiple hyperpigmented skin lesions (café au lait spots) were seen on examination. Plain radiographs showed several 'ground-glass' lesions in the proximal femur and distal tibia. What is the most likely diagnosis?
   a Paget's disease
   b Hand-Schüller-Christian disease
   c Gardner's syndrome
   d Letterer-Siwe disease
   e McCune-Albright syndrome

50 A 25-year-old man presented with a painful leg following a fall playing football. A radiograph showed a pathological fracture of his femur through a well-defined, lytic lesion in the medulla, which was mildly expansile and with a ground-glass matrix. Other than at the fracture there was no disruption of the cortex or soft-tissue mass. What is the most likely diagnosis?
a Fibrous dysplasia
b Metastasis
c Multiple myeloma
d Lymphoma
e Maffucci's syndrome

51 An eight-year-old boy presented with an insidious onset of right-sided shoulder pain. A radiograph showed an aggressive-looking lytic lesion in the metadiaphysis of the proximal humerus. An MRI was subsequently performed, which showed a circumferential extraosseous extension of the tumour with intermediate signal (similar to fat) on T2-weighted images with surrounding oedema. What is the most likely diagnosis?
a Osteomyelitis
b Lymphoma
c Ewing sarcoma
d Acute bone infarction
e Chondroblastoma

52 An X-ray of a 32-year-old gentleman shows a subarticular multiloculated, lytic lesion in the wrist with minimal expansile modelling centred in the metaepiphysis. What is the most likely diagnosis?
a Aneurysmal bone cyst
b Enchondroma
c Intraosseous ganglion
d Unicameral bone cyst
e Giant cell tumour

53 A 66-year-old man presented with a five-month history of back pain. There were no positive findings on examination and a series of blood tests were arranged. These showed: WCC 3.7×10^6/mL, haemoglobin 10.3 g/dL, haematocrit 31%, MCV 85 fl, platelets 110×10^6/mL, total protein 85 g/L, albumin 40 g/L. A chest radiograph showed clear lungs but a number of lucencies in the vertebral bodies. A bone marrow biopsy yielded a red jelly-like material. What cell type is it most likely to contain?
a Giant cells
b Fibroblasts
c Plasma cells
d Metastatic renal carcinoma cells
e Osteoblasts

54 A middle-aged female presented with insidious onset of pain in her left ring finger and no history of trauma. A radiograph showed a solitary well-circumscribed, round lytic lesion with cortical expansion in the diaphysis of the middle phalanx. There is no associated soft-tissue mass. What is the most likely diagnosis?

   a Enchondroma
   b Chondrosarcoma
   c Medullary bone infarction
   d Osteoid osteoma
   e Eosinophilic granuloma

55 A 19-year-old man presented with a history of knee pain and swelling aggravated by movement. His blood tests showed a mildly raised white cell count and raised alkaline phosphatase (ALP). A radiograph showed a Codman's triangle at the margin of a soft-tissue mass. What is the most likely diagnosis?

   a Brodie's abscess
   b Osteosarcoma
   c Ewing sarcoma
   d Haematoma
   e Histiocytosis X

56 A 28-year-old gentleman was known to have a lytic lesion in the metaphysis of his proximal tibia and underwent an MRI scan for further assessment. This showed a well-defined lesion with low signal intensity on both T1- and T2-weighted scans. What is the most likely diagnosis?

   a Intraosseus ganglion
   b Clear cell chondrosarcoma
   c Giant cell tumour
   d Solitary subchondral cyst
   e Brodie's abscess

57 An 86-year-old man was admitted to hospital being unable to weight bear and in poor general health. A pelvic radiograph showed multiple well-circumscribed radiolucent lesions in the iliac wings of the pelvis and a well-defined punched out lesion in the left femoral shaft with disuse osteopenia. What is the most likely diagnosis?

   a Metastatic prostatic deposits
   b Multiple myeloma
   c Fibrous dysplasia
   d Chondrosarcoma
   e Simple bone cysts

58 A nine-year-old girl presented with left hip and knee pain. A subtle well-defined radiolucency was visible in the basi-cervical region of the left femur measuring 6 mm and within this lesion there was a smaller dense opacity. Extensive cortical sclerosis was present around the lesion. What is the most likely diagnosis?

   a Osteoblastoma

   b Chronic sclerosing osteomyelitis

   c Foreign body granuloma

   d Subperiosteal haematoma

   e Osteoid osteoma

59 A 34-year-old man with arm pain had a radiograph which showed a permeative lesion in his humerus, which was expansile and associated with a soft-tissue mass and moderate amount of lamellated periosteal reaction. What is the most likely cause?

   a Simple bone cyst

   b Lymphoma of bone

   c Chondroblastoma

   d Multiple myeloma

   e Non-ossifying fibroma

60 A 38-year-old woman presented with neck pain and motor weakness and was found to have a mass at C6-T2, which was ultimately proven to be an ependymoma. In which part of the spinal canal is this lesion most likely to have originated?

   a Vertebral body

   b Extra dural

   c Dural

   d Subdural

   e Intramedullary

61 At what age does a haemangiopericytoma most commonly present?

   a 0–5 years

   b 10–20 years

   c 30–40 years

   d 50–60 years

   e Over 70 years

62 An 18-year-old female presented with hip pain and was found to have a well-defined lesion in her greater trochanter, which was ultimately proven to be a chondroblastoma. What pattern of mineralisation is typical?

   a Normal surrounding bone, no mineralisation in lesion

   b Normal surrounding bone, rings and arcs within lesion

   c Surrounding sclerosis, no mineralisation in lesion

   d Surrounding osteopenia, dense sclerosis within lesion

   e Surrounding osteopenia, popcorn-shaped densities within lesion

63 At what age is an eosinophilic granuloma most likely to present?

a 0–5 years

b 5–10 years

c 10–20 years

d 30–50 years

e Over 50 years

64 A 42-year-old female was found to have an abnormality of T12 on CT. The vertebral body was not expanded but there was a polka dot appearance with small areas of sclerosis. Due to ongoing symptoms she was assessed with an MRI. What signal is this lesion likely to return?

a Low signal on T1-weighted images, low signal on T2-weighted images

b Low signal on T1-weighted images, high signal on T2-weighted images

c Variable signal on T1-weighted images, high signal on T2-weighted images

d High signal on T1-weighted images, low signal on T2-weighted images

e Variable signal on T1-weighted images, low signal on T2-weighted images

65 A 35-year-old man who presented with back pain was investigated and found to have tuberculous spondylitis. What level is most likely to be affected?

a C3

b T4

c T8

d L1

e L5

66 A 12-year-old boy presented with ankle pain and a radiograph showed a metaphyseal lucency with dense surrounding sclerosis with a thin lucent channel extending towards the growth plate. The lesion was thought to be a Brodie's abscess. What is the most likely causative organism?

a *Proteus mirabilis*

b *Escherichia coli*

c *Staphylococcus aureus*

d *Salmonella* species

e *Streptococcus milleri*

67 A child with an absent thumb and hypoplastic radius has also required treatment for a symptomatic arrhythmia and VSD. What is the most likely underlying unifying diagnosis?

a Down syndrome

b Chondroectodermal dysplasia (Ellis-van Creveld syndrome)

c Holt-Oram syndrome

d Hailey-Hailey syndrome

e Marfan syndrome

68 A 37-year-old female presented with anterior knee pain and was investigated with an MRI scan. There was thinning of the cartilage in the patello-femoral joint, but no abnormality in the femoro-tibial joint. What is the most likely diagnosis?

a Septic arthritis

b Osgood-Schlatter disease

c Sinding-Larsen-Johansson disease

d Chondromalacia patella

e Patella dislocation

69 A 70-year-old man presented with shoulder pain and was assessed with ultrasound. He was found to have torn part of his rotator cuff. Which muscle was most likely to have been damaged?

a Deltoid

b Infraspinatous

c Subscapularis

d Supraspinatous

e Teres minor

70 A 37-year-old male had a CT of his pelvis to investigate abdominal pain and was found to have appendicitis. An incidental finding of a 7-mm enostosis (bone island) was made in his ilium. What is the most appropriate follow-up for the enostosis?

a None

b Chemotherapy

c Radiofrequency ablation

d Excision

e Follow up CT in one year

Musculoskeletal and trauma radiology

PAPER 3

1 A 20-year-old Caucasian male presented to his GP with backache. He was known to be HLA-B27 positive. Imaging of the sacroiliac (SI) joints showed bilateral symmetrical features, extensive sclerosis and erosions. Which of the following is the most likely diagnosis?
   a Osteoarthritis
   b Ankylosing spondylitis
   c Osteitis condensans
   d Reiter syndrome
   e Infection

2 An elderly woman has been complaining of pain in her left hip for many months. The GP is eventually persuaded to request a hip X-ray to investigate this further as the pain is far more severe than her 'regular arthritis' pains. The report from the radiologist reads 'flattening and collapse of left femoral head consistent with avascular necrosis'. Which of the following is the most sensitive in diagnosing avascular necrosis (AVN) of the hip?
   a Bone marrow imaging with radiocolloid
   b Bone scan with diphosphonates
   c Plain films
   d MRI
   e CT

3 An 18-year-old male of African origin with known sickle cell disease presents to the Emergency Department with severe pain in his right thigh. The pain started suddenly two days ago and has not settled with simple analgesics. Plain radiographs are performed which reveal a bone infarct. What appearance would be expected at this time?
   a Increased uptake on the bone scan
   b Sclerosis
   c Calcification
   d Diminished uptake in medullary RES
   e Radiographic changes without cortical involvement

4   A 50-year-old man presented with back pain and subsequent imaging demonstrated flowing ossification of six thoracic vertebral bodies. There was no evidence of ankylosing spondylitis and a diagnosis of diffuse idiopathic skeletal hyperostosis (DISH) was made. What further feature would be most likely on imaging?
    a Ossification of patellar ligament
    b Sclerotic sacroiliac joints
    c Talar osteophytes
    d Fractures of the iliac crest
    e Osteophytes of single vertebral bodies

5   A seven-year-old boy who is known to have Ollier's disease presents with a solid lump close to his knee. What radiological finding is likely?
    a Cartilaginous rest
    b Endosteal reaction
    c Haemangioma
    d Lymphangioma
    e Bony spurs pointing away from the joint

6   A 70-year-old man is known to have histologically confirmed prostate cancer following an ultrasound-guided biopsy a month ago. His PSA has risen to 42 ng/mL and he presents to clinic with increasing lower back pain but no neurology. Which of the following is the single best form of appropriate imaging?
    a Plain film skeletal survey
    b Radionuclide whole body bone scan
    c CT whole spine
    d Contrast enhanced MR of the lumbar spine and pelvis
    e Three-phase radionuclide bone scan of the lumbar spine and pelvis

7   Following acute on chronic back pain a 61-year-old female with a history of steroid use for inflammatory bowel disease is referred for further investigation. Her pelvic and lumbar spine radiographs are unremarkable. An MRI shows patchy low signal in the first sacral segment with loss of height and a radionuclide bone scan shows sacral uptake in an 'h-shaped configuration' with mild degenerative changes elsewhere. What is likely diagnosis based on the above findings?
    a Metastatic deposit
    b Haemangioma
    c Schmorl's node
    d Osteoporotic collapse
    e Insufficiency fracture

8 A 74-year-old man with gout presented with recurrent foot pain and an X-ray of both his feet was taken. What is a typical feature of a joint affected by gout?

a Joint space preserved until late in disease

b No joint effusion

c Periarticular demineralisation

d Erosions with thick sclerotic margins

e Chondrocalcinosis in the majority of cases

9 A 67-year-old man complains of pain in both wrists and ankles. The general practitioner discovers clubbing on digital examination. Plain radiographs are requested, which show changes consistent with hypertrophic osteoarthropathy (HOA). What is the most likely underlying finding in this patient?

a Adrenal adenoma

b Glioblastoma

c Thyroid carcinoma

d Nephroblastoma

e Bronchiectasis

10 A 50-year-old man is known to have haemochromatosis and presents with pain in his hands. What finding would be typical?

a Osteosclerosis

b Geodes

c Chondrocalcinosis

d Asymmetric joint space narrowing

e Narrowing of metacarpal heads

11 A 13-year-old boy presented to his GP with loss of appetite, vomiting, constipation and abdominal pain. His conjunctival membranes were pale. Plain radiographs showed bands of increased density at metaphyses of tubular bones and a 'bone in bone' appearance. Which of the following is most likely to be the cause of these symptoms and findings?

a Active rickets

b Lead poisoning

c Zinc poisoning

d Kennedy disease

e Organic solvent poisoning

12 A 30-year-old patient with no family history of joint or connective tissue disease presented with a stiff leg. X-rays revealed flowing ossification within a dermatomal distribution. What is a further feature of this condition?

a It is caused by Epstein-Barr virus

b It generally does not cross joints

c Extension contractures of the knee

d Rapid course in adults

e Fibrosis of overlying skin is typical

13 A 60-year-old patient with a long history of diabetes peripheral neuropathy presented with ankle deformity. What feature would be in keeping with a Charcot joint?
a Juxta-articular osteoporosis
b Loose bodies
c Severe pain
d Blunted shape of metatarsal heads
e Widened joint space

14 A 14-year-old boy presents to his GP with joint pain, fever, rash and lymphadenopathy. Radiographs showed: rectangular phalanges in the hands and ribbon ribs, pleural effusion and pericardial effusion. What is the most likely diagnosis?
a Osteoarthritis
b Still disease
c Reiter's disease
d Felty's syndrome
e Psoriatic arthritis

15 A 60-year-old patient with hip pain was assessed with a radiograph of their pelvis. Small lucent lines at right angles to the cortex on the medial border of the proximal femoral shaft were visible bilaterally. What would be the most likely underlying diagnosis?
a Osteoporosis
b Fibrous dysplasia
c Hyperthyroidism
d Intraosseous desmoid
e Achondroplasia

16 A middle-aged man presented to the Emergency Department with right hip pain that had started suddenly a few weeks previously and resulted in decreased range of movement. Plain films showed osteoporosis of the hip joint and loss of the subchondral cortex of the femoral head with preservation of the joint space. What is the most likely diagnosis?
a Avascular necrosis
b Transient osteoporosis
c Synovial chondromatosis
d Disuse atrophy
e Villonodular synovitis

17 An overweight 13-year-old boy presented with hip pain. He gave no history of trauma and a radiograph showed widening and irregularity of the capital femoral epiphysis. Several weeks later he represented with worsening symptoms and a repeat radiograph showed displacement of the femoral head. In what direction is it likely the femoral head has displaced?

a Anteroinferior
b Anterolateral
c Anterosuperior
d Posterolateral
e Posteromedial

18 An 18-year-old male with a skin rash on his face had a history of a left knee injury. He had a plain film of his skull to exclude a metal foreign body prior to an MRI scan of his leg, which showed multiple sclerotic lesions in the skull. Films of his initial presentation with his knee injury a year previously showed similar sclerotic lesions with a periosteal reaction in the long bones of his leg and cystic lesions in the distal phalanges of his foot. What is the most likely diagnosis?

a Achondroplasia
b Tuberous sclerosis
c Von Hippel-Lindau syndrome
d Psoriatic arthritis
e Marfan syndrome

19 An 18-year-old boy presented with foot pain and was diagnosed with a talocalcaneal coalition. What sort of coalition is most likely?

a Bony union across anterior facet
b Fibrous coalition across anterior facet
c Bony union across middle facet
d Fibrous coalition across middle facet
e Fibrous union across posterior facet

20 A 46-year-old man presented with back pain and was noted to have marked calcification and loss of height of multiple intervertebral discs, predominately in the lumbar spine. A previous radiograph of his knee also demonstrated premature osteoarthritic changes with pronounced chondrocalcinosis. What is the most likely diagnosis?

a Ankylosing spondylosis
b Ochronosis
c Hyperparathyroidism
d Wilson's disease
e Reiter's syndrome

21 A 67-year-old woman with back pain is investigated with an MRI scan and areas of increased bone marrow signal on T2-weighted images are noted. What is a possible cause?

a Multiple myeloma after treatment
b Lymphoma
c Gaucher's disease
d Radiotherapy
e Sclerotic metastases

22 A 65-year-old lady sustained an injury to her left loin by falling down a flight of stairs. She had a short hypotensive episode but responded well to IV fluids. She was noted to have bruising and severe pain in her loin extending to her back and a urine dipstick showed the presence of microscopic haematuria. What would be the best investigation?
a Observation, no imaging required at present
b Intravenous urogram
c Contrast-enhanced CT
d Ultrasound
e Renal angiogram

23 A 32-year-old motorcyclist presented with blood at the urethral meatus. What is the most effective examination to exclude urethral trauma?
a Multi detector CT
b Pelvic angiography
c MRI
d Retrograde urethrography
e Ultrasound

24 A young girl attended the Emergency Department after tripping over and falling onto her outstretched hand. Clinical examination revealed bruising and swelling on the palmar surface of her hand and she was exquisitely tender in the 'anatomical snuff box'. What would be the best investigation to exclude a scaphoid fracture?
a Immediate plain radiography including scaphoid views
b Plain radiography including scaphoid views after 10 days
c Bone scan within 24 hours
d MRI within 24 hours
e Unenhanced CT

25 An elderly man on warfarin treatment for atrial fibrillation is found at the bottom of a flight of 10 stairs with widespread bruising to his arms and face. On transfer to the Emergency Department he was confused but is otherwise neurologically intact, moving all four limbs and opening his eyes spontaneously. What is the most appropriate investigation?
a Carotid Doppler
b Urgent CT head
c Echocardiogram
d Chest X-ray
e Skull X-ray

26 A 10-year-old boy fell off a climbing frame onto the ground and injured his left elbow. He was assessed in the Emergency Department, and AP and lateral radiographs of his elbow were taken. What finding would be indicative of a fracture?
   a The anterior humeral line passing through the middle third of the capitellum on a lateral view
   b Non-visualisation of the lateral epicondyle
   c Visible anterior fat pad
   d Visible posterior fat pad
   e The radiocapitellar line intersecting the centre of the capitellum

27 An elderly woman tripped on the edge of the curb and fell to the ground. She prevented herself from hitting her head by putting her right hand out in front of her. Her past history was unremarkable other than osteoporosis diagnosed on a DEXA scan two years previously. Immediately after the injury she noticed pain and restricted movement in her right arm. What injury is most likely to be visible on radiographs of the humerus and shoulder?
   a Supracondylar fracture of humerus
   b Posterior dislocation of shoulder joint
   c Fracture of anatomical neck of humerus
   d Fracture of deltoid tuberosity of humerus
   e Fracture of surgical neck of humerus

28 An 18-month-old child presents to the Emergency Department with abdominal pain and her father gives the history that she fell while running. Examination reveals a distressed child with widespread bruises of different ages. Non-accidental injury (NAI) is suspected and a skeletal survey is performed. What injury is most suspicious for NAI?
   a Spiral fracture of the tibia
   b Fracture of left seventh rib posteriorly
   c Greenstick fracture of ulna
   d Supracondylar fracture of the humerus
   e Torus fracture of the radius

29 A 48-year-old female complained of pain in the ulnar aspect of her wrist with no specific antecedent history. Examination did not elicit any positive findings and she was referred for an MRI of her wrist. The only significant finding was a linear band of high signal in a structure just distal to the ulnar styloid that was otherwise of uniformly low signal on both T1- and T2-weighted images. What structure is most likely to have been damaged?
   a Triquetral bone
   b Triangular fibrocartilage
   c Extensor carpi ulnaris tendon sheath
   d Luno-triquetral ligament
   e Proximal surface of lunate bone

30 A 19-year-old hockey player self-referred for physiotherapy for treatment of a long-standing knee problem. A recent radiograph had been reported: 'There is flattening and cortical irregularity of the lateral surface of the medial femoral condyles bilaterally. Subchondral cysts and subchondral sclerosis are present, more marked on the right side.' What is the most likely diagnosis?

   a Osgood-Schlatter disease
   b Osteoarthritis
   c Juvenile chronic arthritis
   d Psoriatic arthritis
   e Osteochondritis dissecans

31 A six-year-old boy fell from a swing onto his outstretched hand. He was reluctant to use his right arm and complained of pain. A radiograph of the right radius and ulna was performed. What is the most likely abnormality?

   a Comminuted fracture of distal radius
   b Pronator quadratus sign
   c Monteggia fracture-dislocation
   d Torus fracture of distal third of the radius
   e Salter-Harris type III fracture of distal radial epiphysis

32 A 62-year-old man was involved in a road traffic accident. There was obvious bruising to the left side of his abdomen and urinalysis revealed microscopic haematuria. There was a delay in obtaining a CT due to a problem with the scanner and a FAST ultrasound examination was performed. What are FAST ultrasound studies able to detect?

   a In the absence of a full bladder FAST can assess for pelvic free fluid
   b 10 mL of ascitic fluid can be reliably detected
   c There is a sensitivity of 40% for the detection of solid-organ injuries
   d FAST scanning is solely for the evaluation of abdominal and pelvic pathology
   e There is a specificity of 70% for mesenteric injuries

33 A 44-year-old back-seat passenger who was restrained with a lap seatbelt was involved in a high-speed road traffic accident. He complained of back pain and after full assessment was found to have a vertebral fracture. A CT scan of his abdomen revealed no intra-abdominal injuries. What is the most likely level of the fracture?

   a C7
   b T2
   c T6
   d L1
   e L4

34 A 45-year-old man with knee pain and instability after a ski injury is assessed in the Orthopaedic Clinic. Clinical examination reveals anterior knee instability with a positive anterior drawer and McMurray test. There is slight crepitus and joint line tenderness. AP and lateral radiographs of the knee are performed, which reveal a small bony fragment just lateral to the lateral tibial plateau. What is the most likely combination of findings?
a Medial meniscus and anterior cruciate ligament tear
b Lateral meniscus and anterior cruciate ligament tear and reverse Segond fracture
c Posterior cruciate ligament and joint capsule tears
d Sesamoid bone in biceps femoris tendon and ligamentous injuries
e Medial meniscus, anterior cruciate ligament tear and Segond fracture

35 A teenager was brought to the Emergency Department after feeling the sensation of his right shoulder 'popping out'. He was unable to use his right arm and radiographs confirmed an anterior dislocation. Which nerve should be specifically examined to exclude an associated injury?
a Musculocutaneous nerve
b Lateral plantar nerve
c Dorsal scapular nerve
d Radial nerve
e Axillary nerve

36 An 83-year-old man was admitted to hospital with a chest infection. Blood tests showed a markedly elevated serum alkaline phosphatase, low albumin, elevated calcium and reduced phosphate. A radiograph of his lumbar spine showed multiple poorly defined sclerotic lesions. What is the most likely underlying diagnosis?
a Fibrous dysplasia
b Ewing sarcoma
c Osteomalacia
d Osteochondromatosis
e Prostate carcinoma

37 A 43-year-old gentleman presented with hyperglycaemia and left-sided chest pain over a period of four months. A radiograph of his chest demonstrated a mass centred on a rib destroying the overlying cortex and associated with a soft-tissue mass. The hyperglycaemia was investigated and felt to be a paraneoplastic phenomenon. What is the most likely diagnosis?
a Adamantinoma
b Chondrosarcoma
c Osteosarcoma
d Myeloma
e Ewing sarcoma

38 A 30-year-old man is found to have an incidental abnormality in his distal femur after a radiograph was performed to investigate a skiing injury. This is a 4-cm well-defined lucent lesion at the lateral margin of the distal end of the femur abutting the articular surface without expansion. What is the most likely diagnosis?
a Aneurysmal bone cyst
b Enchondroma
c Osteoblastoma
d Giant cell tumour
e Osteochondroma

39 A 33-year-old previously healthy man presented with a two-month history of bone pain and headaches. Blood tests show a serum calcium of 13.2 mg/dL with phosphate of 0.6 mM (reference ranges: calcium 8.5–10.5 mg/dL, phosphate 0.8–1.5 mM). Which of the following bone lesions is most frequently associated with these findings?
a Osteitis fibrosa cystica
b Fibrous dysplasia
c Osteochondroma
d Paget's disease of bone
e Giant cell tumour

40 A 24-year-old university student is awaiting treatment of a chondromyxoid fibroma in his proximal tibia when he presents to a different hospital with an incidental injury to his leg. No fracture is visible but what is the expected appearance of this tumour?
a Well-defined lucent lesion with a non-sclerotic margin in the epiphysis
b Well-defined lucent lesion with sclerotic rim in the metaphysis
c Poorly defined lucent lesion in the diaphysis
d Poorly defined lucent lesion in the epiphysis
e Poorly defined lucent lesion in the metaphysis

41 A 19-year-old female presented with lower back pain and a lumbosacral X-ray showed an expansile lytic lesion in the right sacrum. The margins were well defined and there was no soft-tissue mass visible. No other lesions were suspected. What is the most likely diagnosis?
a Multiple myeloma
b Osteoid osteoma
c Chordoma
d Giant cell tumour
e Aneurysmal bone cyst

42 A 25-year-old man was found to have a giant cell tumour in his tibia. What location in the bone is most typical?

a Epiphyseal
b Epiphyseal and metaphyseal
c Metaphyseal
d Metaphyseal and diaphyseal
e Diaphyseal

43 A 73-year-old male with a history of Paget's disease presented with insidious onset low back pain and was assessed with radiographs and MRI, CT and bone scans. Radiographs showed a mixed lytic/sclerotic appearance in the sacrum and an MRI showed infiltration of all five sacral segments with additional anterior soft-tissue extension. There was evidence of osteoid mineralisation within this mass on CT. A bone scan showed these were the only hotspots. What is the most likely diagnosis?

a Sclerotic metastasis
b Lymphoma
c Ewing sarcoma
d Osteoblastoma
e Osteosarcoma

44 A 22-year-old male with an osteosarcoma of his tibia underwent a staging CT which demonstrated a small nodule in his left lower lobe that was thought to represent a metastasis. What is the prognosis for patients with this clinical picture?

(Options given as percentage surviving five years from diagnosis)

a 60–80%
b 40–50%
c 30–40%
d 20–30%
e 10–20%

45 A 20-year-old man slowly developed predominantly nocturnal low back pain. He reports that salicylate-based medication is particularly helpful in relieving his pain. What is the most likely diagnosis?

a Fibrosarcoma
b Malignant fibrous histiocytoma
c Osteoid osteoma
d Chondrosarcoma
e Ollier's disease

46 A man attended a physiotherapy clinic for treatment of long-standing lower back pain. There is no history of trauma and the physiotherapist noted that the patient was systemically well. As he was not improving, a radiograph was requested, which showed a lesion in L4. Which feature would support the diagnosis of an osteoblastoma over another diagnosis?

a Location in the posterior elements
b Patient age under 30
c Absence of a sclerotic rim
d Less than 2-cm diameter
e Cortical disruption

47 An 11-year-old boy presented with left-sided groin pain and recent weight loss. He had been finding it particularly difficult getting in and out of the car when going to school. His mother had been giving him aspirin that helped initially but this no longer had much of an effect. Plain radiographs revealed a 9-mm well-circumscribed lesion with a sclerotic border and central radiolucent nidus within the femoral neck. What is the most likely diagnosis?

a Aneurysmal bone cyst
b Fibrous dysplasia
c Stress fracture of the femoral neck
d Brodie's abscess
e Osteoid osteoma

48 A 34-year-old man presented with a two-month history of pain in his right knee. On examination his right knee was enlarged and tender. A radiograph showed a 9-cm lytic lesion in the epiphysis of the distal femur with a 'soap bubble' appearance. A biopsy showed multinucleated cells in a stroma with spindle-shaped mononuclear cells. What is the most likely diagnosis?

a Tuberculosis
b Giant cell tumour
c Osteosarcoma
d Chondrosarcoma
e Malignant fibrous histiocytoma

49 A bone scan of a 17 year old shows a 'double-density' sign in the femoral neck with a focal centralised region of intense activity surrounded by a region of lesser activity. What is the most likely cause?

a Brodie's abscess
b Simple bone cyst
c Bone infarction
d Osteoid osteoma
e Stress fracture of femoral neck

50 A patient with a known area of fibrous dysplasia in their femur subsequently presented with a soft tissue mass in their thigh and an MRI was arranged. The mass was of low signal on T1- and high signal on T2-weighted images and a biopsy showed it to be a myxoma. What is the likely diagnosis?
a Mazabraud's syndrome
b Ollier's syndrome
c Maffucci's syndrome
d Metastatic malignancy
e Gardner's syndrome

51 Based on age alone, what is the most likely primary bone tumour in a 45-year-old male?
a Osteosarcoma
b Chondrosarcoma
c Giant cell tumour
d Aneurysmal bone cyst
e Osteoid osteoma

52 A 15-year-old boy was recently diagnosed with Ewing sarcoma. What is the most likely bone to be affected?
a Femur
b Humerus
c Sacrum
d Scapula
e Tibia

53 A 14-year-old girl was recently diagnosed with a Ewing sarcoma of her left femur. Which part of the bone is most likely to be affected?
a Epiphyseal
b Epiphyseal and metaphyseal
c Metaphyseal
d Metaphyseal and diaphyseal
e Diaphyseal

54 A 16-year-old boy noticed pain in his knee during his weekly football practice, which was gradually increasing in severity over months. A radiograph showed an aggressive lesion causing a moth-eaten appearance of bone destruction and an associated soft-tissue mass centred on the distal femur. What is the most likely diagnosis?
a Chondrosarcoma
b Metastasis
c Osteochondroma
d Osteogenic sarcoma
e Synovial sarcoma

55 A six-year-old boy was brought to the Emergency Department after falling from a climbing frame. A radiograph showed a fallen fragment within a well-defined unilocular lesion in the proximal humeral metaphysis. There was cortical thinning but no periosteal reaction. What is the most likely underlying diagnosis?

a Osteitis deformans

b Engelmann's disease

c Fibrous dysplasia

d Simple bone cyst

e Osteoid osteoma

56 A radiograph of a 16 year old shows a well-defined lytic lesion with a thin sclerotic margin in the epiphysis of the proximal tibia. On MRI, STIR and T2-weighted images demonstrate a high signal, lobulated lesion with a thin low signal margin. Extensive surrounding bone oedema is seen. What is the most likely diagnosis?

a Aneurysmal bone cyst

b Giant cell tumour

c Chondrosarcoma

d Chondroblastoma

e Brodie's abscess

57 A 15-year-old patient felt a lump on their hand and a radiograph demonstrated an enchondroma. From which part of the bone do enchondromas develop?

a Epiphysis

b Epiphysis and metaphysis

c Metaphysis

d Metaphysis and diaphysis

e Diaphysis

58 A female neonate was born prematurely after a pregnancy complicated by polyhydramnios. A USS of the sacral region demonstrated an 18-cm solid cystic mass and pelvic X-ray demonstrated a mass with amorphous calcification. What blood test would be most helpful in making the diagnosis?

a Beta HCG

b Full blood count

c Alpha feta protein

d Liver function tests

e Urea and electrolytes

59 A 55-year-old man had a history of renal cell carcinoma treated with a radical nephrectomy 10 months previously (T4N1M0). He was thought to be in remission but developed bony pain in his lumbar spine. Lumbar radiographs revealed an abnormality that showed increased uptake on a subsequent Tc-99MDP bone scan. What is the most likely appearance of this lesion on the plain film?

   a Expansile, lytic lesion
   b Non-expansile, lytic lesion
   c Expansile, sclerotic lesion
   d Non-expansile sclerotic lesion
   e Non-expansile, mixed sclerotic/lytic lesion

60 A 29-year-old male presented with difficulty walking and was found to have a complex sensory deficit. After investigation he was found to have an astrocytoma of the spinal cord. Which area is most likely to be involved?

   a Brainstem
   b Cervical spine
   c Thoracic spine
   d Lumbar spine
   e Sacrum

61 A 23-year-old man was investigated with an MRI scan for knee symptoms following an injury playing football four weeks before. On the sagittal images the posterior cruciate ligament was intact but followed an obviously curved course. What underlying injury is likely?

   a None – normal variant
   b Anterior cruciate ligament tear
   c Patella tendon tear
   d Lateral collateral ligament tear
   e Medial collateral ligament tear

62 Where in the body are enchondroma most likely to occur?

   a Femur
   b Humerus
   c Metacarpals
   d Ribs
   e Tibia

63 At what age is an osteoid osteoma most likely to present?

   a 0–10 years
   b 10–30 years
   c 30–50 years
   d 50–70 years
   e Over 70 years

64 A gentleman presented with early onset arthritis and generalised osteoporosis. His hands were worst affected with enlargement of the metacarpal head and loss of joint space particularly in the second and third metacarpophalangeal joints. Which malignancy is he at highest risk of?

a Non-small-cell lung cancer

b Testicular teratoma

c Hepatoma

d Colonic carcinoma

e Melanoma

65 A patient, a keen cross-country runner, was investigated for shin pain and plain radiographs appeared normal. The attending doctor was concerned they may have an occult stress fracture. Which investigation would be most sensitive?

a Repeat plain films after one week

b CT scan

c MRI scan

d Triple phase Tc99m methylene-diphosphonate (MDP) bone scan

e Gallium-67 white cell scan

66 A 40-year-old woman presented with a long history of a painful joint and was found to have pigmented villonodular synovitis (PVNS). Which joint was most likely to have been affected?

a Ankle

b Elbow

c Hip

d Knee

e Shoulder

67 An active 22-year-old man presented with shoulder pain following an injury playing rugby. He was found to have an anterior dislocation of his glenohumeral joint. What associated injury to the glenoid labrum is likely?

a Hill-Sachs lesion

b Reverse Hill-Sachs defect

c Bankart lesion

d Reverse Bankart lesion

e SLAP (Superior labral anterior to posterior) lesion

68 A child with obvious leg length discrepancy was found to have proximal focal femoral deficiency. What other structure(s) is often absent?

a Corpus callosum

b Ossicles

c Cochlea

d Patella

e Clavicles

69 A 15-year-old boy presented with premature ageing and was of short stature. His skin and muscles began to atrophy and he developed diabetes. A chest radiograph showed resorption of the lateral portions of the clavicles and the chest was narrow with thin ribs. He eventually died of a myocardial infarction at 29 years of age. What is the likely inheritance of his condition?

a X-linked recessive

b X-linked dominant

c Mitochondrial

d Autosomal recessive

e Autosomal dominant

70 A 15-year-old athlete presented with pain in the left side of their pelvis and was noted to have a flake of bone adjacent to the anterior inferior iliac spine on their radiograph, which corresponded to the area of tenderness. What muscle are they likely to have avulsed?

a Adductor magnus

b Gracilis

c Psoas

d Rectus femoris

e Sartorius

Gastrointestinal and hepatobiliary radiology

PAPER 1

1   A 54-year-old female presented with dysphagia and an endoscopy was unsuccessful due to a pharyngeal pouch, hence a barium swallow was performed. This showed a mass-like filling defect in the mid third of the oesophagus. A CT showed a focal oesophageal wall mass and histology was obtained, which was consistent with metastatic disease from a distant primary. What is the most likely site of the primary?
    a   Breast
    b   Colon
    c   Hepatic
    d   Ovarian
    e   Pancreas

2   A middle-aged woman presented with reflux and underwent a barium swallow. There was an incidental finding in the cervical oesophagus near the cricopharyngeus where a thin membrane of uniform thickness (2 mm) extending from the anterior oesophageal wall was visible. Her past medical history includes treated hypothyroidism and investigations for iron deficiency anaemia. What is the most likely diagnosis?
    a   Complications related to hypothyroidism
    b   Epidermolysis
    c   Oesophageal stricture
    d   Plummer-Vinson syndrome
    e   Schatzki ring

3   An oral cholecystogram was requested for a patient who had suspected obstruction of the cystic duct. When reviewing the patient's history what is the most definite contraindication to the technique that should be excluded?
    a   Peritonitis
    b   Serious liver disease
    c   Post-operative ileus
    d   Acute pancreatitis
    e   History of atopy

4 A 40-year-old patient presented with right-sided lower abdominal pain. A CT was performed which showed a small pedunculated oval-shaped mass of –60 HU with a more dense peripheral rim and fat stranding adjacent to the proximal descending colon. What is the most likely diagnosis?
a Acute appendicitis
b Perforated appendix with abscess
c Epiploic appendagitis
d Appendiceal tumour
e Diverticulitis

5 An immunocompromised patient with HIV presented acutely with odynophagia. Particularly severe substernal chest pain occurred during swallowing. A double contrast barium swallow was performed which showed multiple small (<1 cm) superficial ulcers in the upper and mid oesophagus without plaque formation. These ulcers had a punctate configuration and were surrounded by radiolucent mounds of oedema. On the basis of the radiological findings what is the most likely diagnosis?
a *Candida* oesophagitis
b CMV oesophagitis
c Herpes oesophagitis
d HIV oesophagitis
e Tuberculous oesophagitis

6 A 32-year-old female was investigated for severe odynophagia with a barium swallow which reproduced the patient's symptoms. The findings were recorded as 'compartmentalisation of the oesophagus with numerous tertiary contractions'. Very high pressures were noted on manometry studies. What is the most likely diagnosis?
a Achalasia
b Chalasia
c Diffuse oesophageal spasm
d Presbyesophagus
e Plummer-Vinson syndrome

7 A patient presented with dysphagia initially to liquids then also gradually to solids. A barium swallow demonstrated a stricture of the distal oesophagus and a subsequent biopsy confirmed malignancy. What cell type would be most likely?
a Lymphoma
b Metastases
c Squamous cell carcinoma
d Leiomyosarcoma
e Adenocarcinoma

8 A 46-year-old female underwent a barium swallow to investigate dysphagia. An indentation was seen on the posterior aspect of the mid thoracic oesophagus. What is the most likely explanation?

a Aberrant left subclavian artery
b Aberrant right subclavian artery
c Normal aortic indentation
d Oesophageal web
e Impression of the cricopharyngeus

9 A 62-year-old woman presented with dysphagia. She was otherwise well but was known to have long-standing diabetes. A barium swallow was performed which showed multiple tiny collections of barium adjacent to the oesophageal lumen. A short distal oesophageal stricture was also noted. With what diagnosis are these radiological findings most consistent?

a Adenomyomatosis
b Erosive oesophagitis
c Oesophageal intramural pseudodiverticulosis
d Pharyngeal pouch
e True oesophageal diverticulum

10 A 21-year-old woman with a long history of recurrent episodes of aspiration pneumonia was noted to have a fluid level within the mediastinum on her chest radiograph. A barium swallow was then performed which showed absence of primary peristalsis and evidence of non-peristaltic contractions. What is the most likely diagnosis?

a Chagas disease
b Peptic stricture
c Primary achalasia
d Scleroderma
e Secondary achalasia

11 A patient presented to the Emergency Department with epigastric and retrosternal pain. A significant oesophageal injury was suspected clinically. Which of the following clinical, radiological or surgical findings are more suggestive of Boerhaave's syndrome than a Mallory-Weiss tear?

a Distal oesophageal injury
b Haematemesis
c History of alcoholism
d Oesophageal mucosal irregularity
e Pneumomediastinum

12 A 12-year-old female child presented with intermittent abdominal pain and vomiting over a two-month period with no weight loss. On examination there was voluntary guarding in the central abdomen but no peritonism. Their inflammatory markers were raised. An ultrasound showed a trace of fluid but no structural abnormality. A technetium-99m pertechnetate scan showed uptake in the stomach and right iliac fossa on the 20-minute images. What is the most likely diagnosis?

a Crohn's disease with multiple sites of activity
b Appendicitis
c Meckel's diverticulum
d Mesenteric adenitis
e Right ovarian torsion

13 A staging CT was performed on a 49-year-old gentleman with a histologically proven adenocarcinoma of the fundus of his stomach. The CT showed invasion of the adjacent contiguous structures but no invasion of adjacent organs, the diaphragm or the abdominal wall. Multiple prominent local nodes were evident and a 1.3-cm (short axis) lymph node was seen in the left para-aortic region. No distant metastases were visible. What is the radiological staging?

a T4b N2 M0
b T4a N3 M0
c T3 N3 M0
d T3 N3 M1
e T4a N2 M0

14 A six-week-old male infant presented with non-bilious projectile vomiting for several days. The baby was dehydrated and found to have a significant electrolyte disturbance. His fontanelles were sunken and a small olive-shaped mass was felt in the upper abdomen. What finding would be expected on ultrasound?

a Delayed gastric emptying
b Exaggerated peristaltic waves
c Pyloric canal length 16 mm; pyloric muscle wall thickness 2 mm
d Pyloric transverse diameter 15 mm and presence of the cervix sign
e Pyloric volume 1.3 cu cm and presence of target lesion sign

15 A patient had recently been diagnosed with gastric carcinoma that had been staged locally as T2 disease. To what extend has the tumour penetrated through the wall?

a Penetrated thorough the serosa
b Invading adjacent organs
c Limited to the submucosa
d Limited to the serosa
e Limited to the mucosa

16 An 80-year-old male underwent a barium meal to investigate epigastric pain and early satiety. There was a narrow, tubular stomach with a lack of rugal folds in the proximal stomach and a smooth greater curve. What is the most likely diagnosis?
   a Zollinger-Ellison syndrome
   b Linitis plastica
   c Atrophic gastritis
   d Menetrier's disease
   e Corrosive gastritis

17 A patient was found unconscious with external signs of abdominal trauma. A CT of their abdomen demonstrated an abnormality around the duodenum with surrounding fluid and further free fluid in the pelvis. The fluid surrounding the duodenum had a measured density of 80 HU. What is this measured area most likely to represent?
   a Active bleeding
   b Fresh unclotted blood
   c Clotted blood
   d Urine
   e Bile

18 A 24 year old developed crampy abdominal pain and diarrhoea over the course of several months and lost a significant amount of weight. He was reluctant to undergo endoscopy and was referred for a barium meal which showed narrowing of the gastric antrum and a cobblestone appearance of the gastric and duodenal mucosa. What is the most likely diagnosis?
   a Crohn's disease
   b Submucosal metastases
   c Zollinger-Ellison syndrome
   d Erosive gastritis
   e Gastric carcinoma

19 A middle-aged man underwent a barium meal which showed an abnormality of the gastric wall with mural thickening, irregularity, reduced distensibility and absent peristalsis. What is the most likely underlying diagnosis?
   a Amyloid
   b Pancreatic carcinoma
   c Radiation therapy
   d Scirrhous cancer
   e Syphilis

20 An 80-year-old man was readmitted to the surgical ward one month after an elective abdominal aortic aneurysm repair complaining of nausea and vomiting. A plain abdominal radiograph demonstrated gaseous distension of the stomach and duodenal bulb. Contrast-enhanced CT did not reveal any further abnormality and a barium meal was performed which showed stricturing of the distal duodenum. What is the most likely explanation for these findings?
    a Adhesions
    b Annular pancreas
    c Duodenal haematoma
    d Infected Dacron vascular graft
    e Paralytic ileus

21 A young man was involved in a fight in a fast food outlet and was stabbed in the abdomen with a large knife. A CT of his chest, abdomen and pelvis showed a duodenal laceration with associated pneumoperitoneum and intra-peritoneal free fluid. What other organ is most likely to have been injured?
    a Colon
    b Liver
    c Pancreas
    d Small bowel
    e Spleen

22 A 17-year-old was a rear-seat passenger in a head-on vehicle collision with a combined speed of 120 mph in which the drivers both died at the scene. The patient was wearing a seatbelt and was not ejected from the vehicle. After being cut from the vehicle the patient was airlifted to hospital where a multi-trauma CT was performed. In addition to significant head and chest trauma there was intraperitoneal free fluid and some bubbles of extraluminal intraperitoneal free gas just beyond the ligament of Treitz. There was also duodenal and jejunal wall thickening. What is the most likely diagnosis?
    a Jejunal injury with disruption of the bowel wall
    b Duodenal injury with disruption of the bowel wall
    c Bowel oedema secondary to hypovolaemic shock
    d Blunt injury causing contusion of the jejunum and duodenum
    e Pancreatic contusion

23 An eight-month-old female had been crying inconsolably for 12 hours during which time she had passed at least two bloodstained stools. She was admitted to hospital and a plain abdominal radiograph showed a soft mass in the right upper quadrant which corresponded to a fullness of the abdomen on physical examination. An ultrasound was performed which showed a 'pseudokidney' in this region. What is the most likely diagnosis?
    a Ileocolic intussusception
    b Ileoileocolic intussusception
    c Mid-gut volvulus

d Ileo-ileal intussusception

e Pyloric stenosis

24 A 51-year-old male was investigated for vague abdominal symptoms including abdominal pain and weight loss. Physical examination revealed generalised peripheral lymphadenopathy and some areas of hyperpigmentation of the skin. A diagnosis of Whipple disease was suspected and a small bowel contrast study was performed. What features would most support this diagnosis?

a Sand-like nodules (approx 1 mm) in non-dilated small bowel

b Small nodules (>2 mm) in non-dilated small bowel

c Thick folds in non-dilated small bowel

d Normal folds in dilated small bowel

e Thick folds in dilated small bowel

25 A patient underwent a small bowel follow-through study, which you have been asked to review. The luminal diameter was 2 cm and the valvulae conniventes and wall both measure 1-mm thick. What is the correct conclusion?

a Crohn's disease

b Normal study

c Blind loop syndrome

d Small bowel obstruction

e Small bowel lymphoma

26 A young adult male who had recently moved to the UK from India presented with abdominal pain, diarrhoea and weight loss. A CT showed evidence of ileitis. Stool cultures were negative. What feature would favour a diagnosis of tuberculous ileitis rather than Crohn's disease?

a Aphthous ulcers

b Isolated terminal ileal involvement

c Small rosethorn ulcers

d Thickening of circular small bowel folds

e Ulcers with elevated margins following lymphoid follicles

27 A 26-year-old female presented with a long history of abdominal bloating, pale loose stools and weight loss. She underwent a series of investigations including a small bowel enema and eventually, following jejunal biopsy, was diagnosed with coeliac disease (nontropical sprue). What radiographic features are most likely to have been visible on her small bowel enema?

a Reversal of jejunal and ileal fold patterns

b Stricturing lesions

c Enteroenteric fistulae

d Polypoidal small bowel filling defects

e The moulage sign

28 A patient with known ulcerative colitis was admitted as an emergency. Their plain abdominal radiograph showed dilation and mucosal islands in keeping with toxic megacolon. In which part of the large bowel are these changes most commonly seen?
   a Caecum
   b Ascending colon
   c Transverse colon
   d Descending colon
   e Sigmoid colon

29 A 22-year-old male with severe Crohn's disease had recurring problems with anal fistulae. An MR fistulogram was undertaken and reported 'a tract extends laterally from the rectal mucosa in the region of the dentate line through the internal sphincter and then infero-medially to skirt the medial aspect of the external sphincter and runs to an area 1 cm or so from the anus itself'. What type of fistula is this?
   a Suprasphincteric
   b Extrasphincteric
   c Transsphincteric
   d Intersphincteric
   e Superficial

30 An 80-year-old lady presented with an acute abdomen. She suffered from diabetes, hypercholesterolaemia and had a long smoking history. On examination she has a diffusely tender abdomen with decreased bowel sounds and her pulse was irregularly irregular. Acute mesenteric ischaemia was suspected and a CT was arranged. What feature is most likely to suggest superior mesenteric artery compromise?
   a Mesenteric and portal vein gas
   b Small bowel pseudo-obstruction
   c Gasless abdomen
   d Thumbprinting of bowel wall
   e Bowel distension to the splenic flexure

31 A middle-aged patient with a history of epilepsy (associated with a known supratentorial glioblastoma) underwent an elective colonoscopy and a colorectal carcinoma was identified among multiple colonic polyps that varied in size up to 30 mm. Which is the most likely diagnosis?
   a Familial adenomatous polyposis
   b Peutz-Jeghers
   c Turcot syndrome
   d Gardner
   e Cowden disease

32 A 60-year-old male presented with change in bowel habit, weight loss and anaemia. Flexible sigmoidoscopy demonstrated a mass in the sigmoid colon and biopsy showed it to be an adenocarcinoma. MRI of the pelvis showed invasion of the muscularis propria and CT showed eight significantly enlarged local pericolic nodes. No further significant lymphadenopathy was present and there were no lung metastases. What radiological staging is most appropriate?

a T1, N0, M1

b T2, N2, M0

c T3, N2, M0

d T4, N0, M0

e T2, N1, M0

33 A 67-year-old female had a CT of her abdomen and pelvis to investigate abdominal pain. This showed a suspicious rectosigmoid lesion, which was subsequently biopsied and found to be adenocarcinoma. What would be the next appropriate imaging?

a Ultrasound liver, CXR, MRI pelvis

b MRI pelvis and CT chest

c MRI pelvis and MRI liver

d CT chest, MRI pelvis and whole body PET

e Whole body PET and MRI pelvis

34 A young female patient with Crohn's disease was due to be assessed for recurrent episodes of perianal sepsis. What is the most appropriate modality for imaging the pelvis?

a Transvaginal ultrasound

b Contrast-enhanced CT of abdomen and pelvis

c PET-CT scan

d MRI pelvis

e Transrectal ultrasound

35 A patient with infectious colitis underwent an abdominal CT scan. Thickening and reduced attenuation of the colonic wall of the right hemicolon was visible. The remainder of the bowel was unremarkable. What causative organism is most likely to account for these radiological findings?

a *Cytomegalovirus* (CMV)

b *Escherichia coli*

c Gonorrhoea

d *Clostridium difficile*

e *Shigella*

36 A 52-year-old man was admitted to the medical high dependency unit with a severe colitis. Routine biochemical, haematological and microbiological specimens were taken and a plain abdominal radiograph and portable abdominal ultrasound were performed. Further enquiry revealed that he had recently been treated with broad spectrum antibiotics, but also has a background of a longer history of colitic symptoms. What radiological features would support a diagnosis of pseudo-membranous colitis rather than ulcerative colitis?

a Arthritis
b Ascites
c Excessive rectosigmoid fat
d Polyp formation
e Pancolitis

37 A diabetic 50-year-old man was investigated for hepatic disease. His liver was enlarged and he had hyperpigmentation of his skin. His serum iron was >300 mg/dL and serum transferrin saturation was >50%. What imaging feature is most characteristic of the underlying diagnosis?

a Increase in hepatic echogenicity on US
b Patchy echogenicity demonstrated on US
c Decrease in hepatic T1 signal on MR
d Decrease in hepatic attenuation on CT
e Decrease in hepatic T2 signal on MR

38 A front-seat passenger in a head-on collision was brought to the Emergency Department. A contrast-enhanced CT of their abdomen and pelvis showed a liver laceration in segment 6 that is 2 cm deep and 8 cm long. What grade is appropriate?

a Grade I laceration
b Grade II laceration
c Grade III laceration
d Grade IV laceration
e Grade V laceration

39 Following a holiday in South-East Asia, a 33-year-old man presented with abdominal pain. Ultrasound demonstrated an echo-poor lesion within the right lobe of the liver which contained several smaller internal cysts. What is the most likely diagnosis?

a Amoebic abscess
b *Echinococcus*
c Pyogenic abscess
d Polycystic liver disease
e Haemangioma

40 A 67-year-old woman noticed an abdominal mass and was referred for an ultrasound scan. This showed a large, uniformly hyperechoic mass in the left lobe of the liver. A subsequent multi-phase contrast-enhanced CT confirmed this mass which enhances peripherally until it becomes isoattenuating with the adjacent liver parenchyma after five minutes. What is the most likely diagnosis?

a Adenoma

b Haemangioma

c Hepatocellular carcinoma

d Focal nodular hyperplasia

e Solitary metastasis

41 A 38-year-old woman presented with upper abdominal discomfort. She was otherwise well and was taking the combined oral contraceptive pill. Physical examination was normal. An ultrasound showed a well-circumscribed, homogeneous 4-cm mass in the liver and she was subsequently referred for a liver MRI. What feature would be most useful in distinguishing focal nodular hyperplasia from adenoma?

a Calcification

b Internal haemorrhage

c Multiple lesions

d Uptake of reticuloendothelial contrast

e Uptake of hepatobiliary contrast

42 A middle-aged man with symptoms of lethargy and painful hands presented to his doctor. Routine blood tests showed deranged liver function and plain radiographs of his hands showed an arthropathy primarily affecting the first and second metacarpophalangeal (MCP) joints. He was referred to a hepatologist and an abdominal CT was arranged. The liver was of diffusely increased density prior to contrast administration. What is the most likely underlying diagnosis?

a Amiodarone treatment

b Glycogen storage disorder

c Haemochromatosis

d Primary biliary cirrhosis

e Rheumatoid arthritis

43 A 58-year-old African woman was visiting her grandchildren in London when she developed right upper quadrant pain. The local doctor, suspecting gallstones, arranged an ultrasound which showed a grossly cirrhotic liver with markedly hyperechoic septa separating areas of relatively normal liver. The scanning radiologist recognised this as a 'turtle back' appearance. What is the most likely underlying diagnosis?

a Amoebiasis

b Hydatid

c Lymphoma

d Schistosomiasis

e Tuberculosis

44 A 17-year-old male developed upper abdominal pain and abdominal distension two days after an appendicectomy. He had been dehydrated on presentation but the operation was uncomplicated. Transabdominal ultrasound showed a large volume of ascites and a diagnosis of portal vein thrombosis was considered. What sonographic finding is most commonly seen that would support this diagnosis?

a Portosystemic collateral circulation
b Increase in portal vein diameter
c Echogenic material in the portal vein lumen
d Enlargement of a thrombosed portal vein above 15 mm
e Enlargement of the lesser omentum

45 A 65-year-old recently retired labourer had an abdominal CT to investigate general malaise. This showed multiple discrete areas of low attenuation within the spleen, which were rounded with ill-defined margins and distorted the splenic contour. It was thought that these were most likely to represent metastatic disease but the primary was not visible on the scan. What is the most likely site of the underlying primary tumour?

a Bronchogenic carcinoma
b Undetected colon carcinoma
c Renal cell carcinoma
d Prostate carcinoma
e Malignant melanoma

46 In a normal adult patient, what is the relative signal intensity of the liver, muscle and spleen on T1-weighted imaging? (Options are presented in order of decreasing signal intensity, i.e. highest signal first.)

a Liver > muscle > spleen
b Liver > spleen > muscle
c Muscle > spleen > liver
d Muscle > liver > spleen
e Spleen > muscle > liver

47 A 45-year-old male with a previous history of a splenectomy post trauma as a child was being assessed to determine if he had splenosis. What is the most sensitive modality?

a Angiography
b Contrast-enhanced CT
c MRI
d Nuclear medicine studies
e Ultrasound

48 A 24-year-old HIV-positive patient presented with vague abdominal pain and fever. Ultrasound of the abdomen demonstrated hepatomegaly and multiple rounded lesions of low reflectivity within the spleen consistent with splenic microabscesses. What is the most likely causative organism?

   a *Cytomegalovirus* (CMV)
   b Fungal
   c *Haemophilus*
   d *Staphylococcus aureus*
   e *Streptococcus pneumoniae*

49 A 62-year-old man was admitted with sepsis and abdominal pain. Contrast-enhanced abdominal CT revealed splenic enlargement and several low-attenuation lesions within the spleen. Subsequent ultrasound-guided aspiration yielded infected material. What is the commonest cause of a splenic abscess?

   a Adjacent pericolic abscess
   b Haematogenous spread
   c Splenic infarction
   d Penetrating trauma
   e Following intervention or surgery

50 Elective CT colonography was performed on an otherwise well 70-year-old gentleman to investigate a recent change in bowel habit and a history of weight loss. Fortunately, no evidence of a colorectal malignancy was identified but there was an incidental finding that the gallbladder was in an unusual position. Where is the most common position for an ectopic gallbladder to lie?

   a Beneath the left lobe of liver
   b Intrahepatic
   c Retrohepatic
   d Within falciform ligament
   e Within interlobar fissure

51 A middle-aged female underwent an ultrasound for right upper quadrant pain. This showed multiple gallstones in a thin-walled gallbladder with no intrahepatic biliary duct dilatation. The common bile duct was not dilated and did not contain any gallstones. What is the likely composition of this patient's gallstones?

   a Calcium
   b Calcium bilirubinate
   c Cholesterol
   d Cysteine
   e Urate

52 A fit 67-year-old female underwent an ultrasound to investigate right upper quadrant pain which demonstrated an abnormal gallbladder. Further imaging with CT confirmed a diagnosis of a porcelain gallbladder. What is the probability of a carcinoma developing in such patients?

a 1%

b 15%

c 50%

d 85%

e 99%

53 A 40-year-old woman was admitted to the Neuro-ITU after a subarachnoid bleed and on day nine developed systemic inflammatory response syndrome (SIRS). She had, by this stage, been successfully weaned off the ventilator and her chest radiograph and urine cultures were normal. Blood cultures grew *Salmonella*. A limited portable transabdominal ultrasound showed free fluid in the upper abdomen. What is the most likely diagnosis?

a Acute pancreatitis

b Perforated peptic ulcer disease

c Portal vein thrombosis

d Acute cholecystitis

e Ruptured abdominal aortic aneurysm

54 A 40-year-old woman underwent transabdominal ultrasound for investigation of right upper quadrant pain two days after an uncomplicated laparoscopic cholecystectomy. This showed a moderate volume of subhepatic free fluid, but a normal common bile duct (CBD). A diagnostic aspirate of this fluid showed it contained bile. What complication is she most likely to have suffered?

a Clipping of the CBD

b Transection of the CBD

c Liver haemorrhage

d Injury to the duct of Luschka

e Subhepatic abscess

55 A patient presented unwell with abdominal pain and bilious vomiting. They had previously suffered from episodes of acute cholecystitis secondary to gallstones. On this occasion initial investigations showed abnormal liver function tests and a plain abdominal radiograph demonstrated an ileus. The surgical team requested a CT as they were concerned of the possibility of a biliary-enteric fistula. A contrast-enhanced abdominal CT was performed and pneumobilia was noted. What other feature would most support the diagnosis of a biliary-enteric fistula?

a Distended gallbladder with a thickened wall up to 5 mm

b Gallbladder totally collapsed around multiple small gallstones

c Shrunken gallbladder mimicking a diverticulum of the duodenal bulb

d Shrunken gallbladder with a thickened wall up to 5 mm

e Thick-walled gallbladder directly adjacent to the duodenal bulb

56 A 23-year-old female with a history of vague upper abdominal pain was investigated with an ultrasound which demonstrated multiple cystic structures converging towards the porta hepatis and communicating with the bile ducts. Cholangiography showed ectactic intrahepatic ducts extending to the periphery and the common bile duct was also dilated. What is the most likely diagnosis?

a Biliary hamartoma
b Caroli's disease
c Primary biliary cirrhosis
d Primary sclerosing cholangitis
e Pyogenic cholangitis

57 A previously well elderly male patient was admitted with painless obstructive jaundice. Upper abdominal ultrasound showed intrahepatic duct dilatation but normal-calibre extrahepatic ducts. Percutaneous transhepatic cholangiography with separate left and right duct system punctures demonstrated dilated but otherwise normal intrahepatic ducts. The central ducts were not opacified. What is the most likely diagnosis?

a Inflammatory biliary stricture
b Klatskin tumour
c Pancreatic head tumour
d Primary biliary cirrhosis
e Primary sclerosing cholangitis

58 A 40-year-old woman with a one-year history of symmetrical metacarpophalangeal joint arthritis and a dry mouth was admitted with abdominal distension. She underwent a contrast-enhanced CT of her liver which showed ascites, marked caudate hypertrophy and scattered dilated intrahepatic ducts. Her common bile duct measured 5 mm. What is the most likely diagnosis?

a Primary sclerosing cholangitis
b Obstructive cholangiolithiasis
c Primary biliary cirrhosis
d Alcoholic hepatitis
e Haemochromatosis

59 A 55-year-old man was investigated for weight loss and jaundice. A contrast-enhanced CT showed dilated intrahepatic biliary ducts, a common bile duct of 12-mm and a pancreatic duct of 3-mm diameter. No causative mass was seen but an ampullary tumour was suspected. What is the most sensitive technique for local staging?

a CT
b Endoscopic ultrasound
c ERCP
d MRCP
e Laparoscopy

60 An 80-year-old man was admitted with epigastric pain. A transabdominal ultrasound revealed two large epigastric cysts which appeared simple, and a contrast-enhanced CT showed them to be intrahepatic cysts occupying the left lobe and associated with marked left lobar atrophy. There was right lobar intrahepatic duct dilatation but the common bile duct was of normal calibre. What should be the next appropriate step in his management?

a No follow-up

b Repeat transabdominal ultrasound in three months

c Interval CT in six months

d MRI liver

e Diagnostic aspiration

61 A two-week-old male neonate was noted to be becoming progressively more jaundiced. Transabdominal ultrasound showed mild hepatomegaly with an echogenic 'triangle' of tissue at the porta hepatis. The gallbladder appeared normal but there was polysplenia. What is the most likely diagnosis?

a Neonatal hepatitis

b Sclerosing cholangitis

c Haemolysis

d Congenital biliary atresia

e Alagille Syndrome

62 A 39-year-old male alcoholic represented to the Emergency Department feeling generally unwell three weeks after an initial diagnosis of acute pancreatitis. He self-discharged himself from hospital after 10 days of treatment. His original CT at diagnosis showed inflammation of the whole gland and a repeat CT on his representation showed a well-demarcated 4 cm × 3 cm fluid collection directly anterior to the body of the pancreas which contained a small bleb of gas. What is the most likely diagnosis?

a Acute pseudocyst

b Enteric fistula

c Gland necrosis

d Pancreatic abscess

e Pancreatic phlegmon

63 A patient with Von Hippel-Lindau syndrome was being investigated for renal symptoms and an incidental finding in the pancreas was made on CT. A 5-cm lobulated mass with the appearance of a 'bunch of grapes' was seen in the neck of the gland. There was a prominent central stellate scar within this lesion and distal dilatation of the pancreatic duct. What is the most likely diagnosis?

a Acinar cell carcinoma

b Intraductal papillary mucinous tumour

c Papillary neoplasm of the pancreas

d Pancreatic ductal adenocarcinoma

e Serous cystadenoma of the pancreas

64 A two-week-old baby with Down syndrome was admitted under the Paediatric team with persistent vomiting. A plain abdominal radiograph demonstrated a double bubble. An ultrasound showed proximal duodenal dilatation and concentric narrowing of the lumen at the second part of the duodenum with a bulky pancreatic head. What diagnosis best fits with these features?
a Annular pancreas
b Duodenal atresia
c Duodenal stenosis
d Malrotation
e Pyloric stenosis

65 CT is more sensitive than MRI for the detection of calcifications associated with chronic pancreatitis but MRI is a useful tool in assessing duct and parenchymal abnormalities in cases of chronic pancreatitis. Which abnormality is most likely to lead to a false negative on MRI?
a Demonstrating dilated duct upstream from an obstruction
b Demonstrating gland atrophy
c Demonstrating intraductal stones
d Evaluating duct strictures
e Demonstrating intraductal stones not surrounded by fluid

66 A pancreatic transplant patient had an ultrasound three weeks after their transplant procedure. It was difficult to delineate the margins of the gland and there was acoustic inhomogeneity and a dilated pancreatic duct. What is the correct interpretation of these features?
a Acute rejection
b Graft vessel thrombosis
c Pancreatitic abscess
d Pancreatitis
e Normal post-procedural appearances

67 A young boy presented after hitting the handlebars of his push bike. Imaging demonstrated pancreatic parenchymal damage that did not involve the main pancreatic duct. What is the most likely site of injury?
a Pancreatic head
b Uncinate process
c Pancreatic tail
d Junction of head and neck
e Junction of body and tail

68 A 23-year-old man with cystic fibrosis underwent a thoracic CT to assess his pulmonary disease. The upper abdomen was included and the pancreas was noted to appear abnormal. What is the most likely pancreatic abnormality?
a Macrocystic change
b 'String-of-pearls' pancreatic duct
c Stranding of the peripancreatic fat
d Pancreas divisium
e Diffuse pancreatic atrophy

69 A 58-year-old man presented with upper abdominal pain, haematemesis and diarrhoea. He had been treated with a proton pump inhibitor for epigastric pain for a year with little effect. Oesophagogastroduodenoscopy (OGD) revealed multiple erosions but no varices and an ultrasound showed a hypoechoic mass in the body of the pancreas. What is the most likely cause of the pancreatic abnormality?
a Adenocarcinoma
b Gastrinoma
c Metastasis
d Pseudocyst
e VIPoma

70 A 50-year-old woman who had been treated for cervical carcinoma 18 months previously presented with colicky abdominal pain. A CT showed thickening of the ileal wall with luminal narrowing, which was causing partial obstruction. There was also increased attenuation of the associated mesentery. What is the most likely diagnosis?
a Carcinoid
b Crohn's disease
c Ischaemic bowel
d Lymphoma
e Radiation enteritis

Gastrointestinal and hepatobiliary radiology

PAPER 2

1   A 53-year-old gentleman was investigated for mild dysphagia. He was found to have an area of focal wall thickening at the junction of the mid and distal thirds of the oesophagus, which was shown to be squamous cell carcinoma on biopsy. After further assessment there was no evidence of distant disease and depending on local staging the patient could be a candidate for aggressive surgery. What would be the modality of choice for accurate local staging?
    a   Dual-phase contrast-enhanced CT of chest, abdomen and pelvis
    b   Endoscopic ultrasound
    c   MRI
    d   PET-CT
    e   Triple-phase contrast-enhanced CT of chest, abdomen and pelvis

2   A 55-year-old male with a history of drug and alcohol abuse underwent an elective barium swallow for follow-up after surgery for laryngeal carcinoma. This demonstrated tortuous longitudinal filling defects in the lower third of a partially collapsed oesophagus. What is the most likely cause of these radiological findings?
    a   Achalasia
    b   Mucosal oedema associated with oesophagitis
    c   Oesophageal lymphoma
    d   Oesophageal varices
    e   Varicoid oesophageal carcinoma

3   An 82-year-old man attended for an outpatient double-contrast barium enema to investigate alteration in bowel habit. When reviewing the patient's history what is the most definite contraindication to the technique that should be excluded?
    a   Rigid endoscope rectal biopsy three days ago
    b   Type 2 diabetes mellitus
    c   Angina
    d   Open-angle glaucoma
    e   Colonic resection two years previously

4   A patient with a history of closed angle glaucoma was due to undergo a barium
     meal and substitution of glucagon for hyoscine-N-butyl bromide (Buscopan®)
     was planned. What would be a contraindication to glucagon use?
     a Iodine allergy
     b Myasthenia gravis
     c Phaeochromocytoma
     d Prostatic enlargement
     e Pyloric stenosis

5   A patient with Parkinson's disease had an elective barium swallow to investig-
     ate symptoms of dysphagia. Which radiological appearance is most consistent
     with the presence of tertiary contractions?
     a Local peristaltic wave elicited through oesophageal distension
     b Local peristaltic wave identical to primary wave
     c Orderly peristaltic sequence
     d Stripping wave clearing the barium
     e 'Yo-Yo' motion of the barium

6   A 47-year-old male inpatient was investigated for vague symptoms of dys-
     phagia. Both an upper gastrointestinal endoscopy study and a barium swallow
     were performed. What appearances most support the diagnosis of scarring
     secondary to reflux oesophagitis?
     a Fixed rigid folds with abrupt demarcation
     b Fixed transverse folds with stepladder appearance of distal oesophagus
     c Longitudinal folds >3 mm with evidence of submucosal inflammation
     d Tortuous folds effaced by oesophageal distension
     e Mass within the oesophageal wall

7   A patient underwent a barium swallow to investigate dysphagia. There was an
     indentation on the anterior aspect of the oesophagus anterior to the C5 ver-
     tebral body. The remainder of the study is unremarkable. What is the most
     likely cause for this appearance?
     a Oesophageal web
     b Cricoid impression
     c Oesophageal diverticulum
     d Oesophageal neoplasm
     e Oesophageal dysmotility

8   A middle-aged man presented with symptoms of epigastric pain worse after
     eating. A diagnosis of Barrett's oesophagus was made. What are the most
     likely histological findings?
     a Columnar epithelium replacing stratified squamous epithelium
     b Stratified squamous epithelium replacing columnar epithelium
     c Transitional cell epithelium replacing stratified squamous epithelium
     d Transitional cell epithelium replacing columnar epithelium
     e Infiltration with adenocarcinoma

9   Following a barium swallow, the reporting radiologist proposes a likely diagnosis of Barrett's oesophagus. Which of the following radiological findings are likely to have supported this diagnosis?
a   A short proximal stricture
b   A long distal stricture
c   An oesophageal diverticulum
d   A large shallow ulcer
e   An extrinsic compressive mass

10   A 60-year-old female patient complained of intermittent episodes of dysphagia to solid foods, which were particularly severe when eating steak. A contrast swallow demonstrated a thin constriction at the gastro-oesophageal junction. The narrowing was smooth, symmetrical and very short (2 mm). What is the most likely diagnosis?
a   Achalasia
b   Barrett's oesophagus
c   Lymphoma
d   Oesophageal carcinoma
e   Schatzki ring

11   A new drug is being evaluated and the results of a placebo controlled trial are published. The primary end point was all cause death and the trial reports that of 400 people studied 20 of the 200 in the treatment arm died and 40 of the 200 in the control group. What is the number needed to treat (NNT) for this drug?
a   0.1
b   2
c   5
d   9
e   10

12   An adult male presented with weight loss and intermittent abdominal pain. A CT demonstrated a small bowel mass and adjacent soft-tissue mesenteric mass with calcification. An In-111 labelled octreotide study was performed with SPECT images which demonstrated uptake in the small bowel and mesenteric mass and further uptake in the liver and lungs. What is the likely diagnosis?
a   Extra adrenal phaeochromocytoma (paraganglioma)
b   Carcinoid syndrome
c   Widespread carcinoid metastases
d   Metastatic gastrointestinal stromal tumour (GIST)
e   Lymphoma

13 An 88-year-old lady presented with a tender distended abdomen. A dilated viscus was visible in the left upper quadrant on plain radiography with a long fluid level. There was leftward and upward displacement with a raised left hemidiaphragm and little gas elsewhere in the abdomen. What is the most likely diagnosis?

a Air swallowing
b Caecal volvulus
c Gastric outlet obstruction
d Gastric volvulus
e Paralytic ileus

14 An eight-year-old girl presented with a month's history of abdominal pain and vomiting. An abdominal ultrasound demonstrated a cyst with an inner echogenic layer and outer hypoechoic layer of muscle in the region of the greater curvature of the stomach. What is the most likely diagnosis?

a Gastric duplication cyst
b Mesenteric cyst
c Oesophageal duplication cyst
d Pancreatic cyst
e Pancreatic pseudocyst

15 A gastric ulcer was visible during a barium meal. What feature would favour a benign aetiology over malignancy?

a Irregular contour
b Hampton's line
c Shallow ulcer
d No protrusion beyond stomach
e Asymmetrical mass

16 A patient was diagnosis with Menetrier's disease on histology. What radiological appearance would support this diagnosis?

a Absence of gastric folds in the proximal stomach
b Thickened folds in the proximal stomach
c Multiple gastric ulcers
d Rigid stomach wall
e Aphthoid ulcers

17 A patient underwent a barium meal which demonstrated multiple filling defects. Upper GI endoscopy confirmed multiple gastric polyps, which were biopsied. What is the histology most likely to show?

a Adenomatous polyps
b Hamartomatous polyps
c Hyperplastic polyps
d Leiomyomas
e Metastases

18 A 50-year-old publican with a history of back pain developed retrosternal pain and melaena. He visited his doctor and, following a negative urea breath test, was referred for a barium meal. This showed linear streaks and dots of barium within the gastric mucosa, preferentially affecting the gastric antrum. What is the most likely diagnosis?

   a Crohn's disease
   b Gastric varices
   c Gastric carcinoma
   d Emphysematous gastritis
   e Erosive gastritis

19 A 30-year-old man with no previous medical or surgical history presented to the Emergency Department with severe epigastric pain. He was retching but was unable to vomit. Plain radiographs demonstrated a large hiatus hernia and grossly distended stomach and an abdominal CT revealed features of a gastric volvulus associated with the hiatus hernia. What feature would suggest an organoaxial volvulus?

   a Diaphragmatic rupture
   b Evidence of gastric ischaemia
   c Gas in the stomach wall
   d Greater curvature located cranially
   e The fundus positioned caudal to the antrum

20 A 17-year-old man with a history of recurrent chest infections developed dysphagia. The patient was not able to tolerate an endoscopy and he was referred for a barium meal. This demonstrated thickened, nodular duodenal mucosal folds. Review of a recent chest radiograph showed bronchiectasis mainly affecting the upper zones. What is the most likely underlying diagnosis?

   a Cystic fibrosis
   b Kartagener syndrome
   c Duodenal lymphoma
   d Scleroderma
   e Tuberculosis

21 A patient presented with anaemia and ongoing melaena. Colonoscopy and blood biochemistry results were normal. Red blood cell scintigraphy localised the source of bleeding to the small bowel and an ultrasound of the abdomen showed a well-defined, spherical mass of low reflectivity measuring 5 cm in diameter. What is the most likely diagnosis?

   a Carcinoid
   b Leiomyoma
   c Lymphoma
   d Adenocarcinoma
   e Tuberculosis

22 An otherwise well 19-year-old male was seen in Gastroenterology Outpatients with a long history of diarrhoea and weight loss. He was noted to have mouth ulcers and a few reddened raised areas on his shins. A small bowel follow-through, colonoscopy and further blood tests were arranged. What is the most likely finding on the follow-through?
   a Linear ulcers on mesenteric border
   b Shallow small rounded ulcers
   c Double tracking ulcers
   d Single large (>5 cm) deep ulcer
   e Mass lesion

23 A 14-year-old boy presented with crampy abdominal pain and a history of darkened stools over the last few weeks. Physical examination was normal other than some vague central abdominal tenderness and pigmentation of the lower lip. An urgent ultrasound showed a probable intussusception. Following reduction a follow-up small bowel study showed multiple broad-based polyps mainly in the jejunum and ileum. What is the most likely diagnosis?
   a Familial adenomatous polyposis
   b Cowden syndrome
   c Juvenile polyposis
   d Cronkhite-Canada syndrome
   e Peutz-Jeghers syndrome

24 An infant presented unwell, was found to have an intussusception and reduction was planned. What is the most suitable technique for reduction?
   a Four attempts at hydrostatic reduction
   b Hydrostatic reduction at 120 mmHg
   c Hydrostatic reduction at 220 mmHg
   d Single attempt at pneumatic reduction for four minutes
   e Two attempts at pneumatic reduction two minutes apart

25 A previously well 55-year-old male presented with diarrhoea, facial flushing and wheeze. After further investigation he was found to have a carcinoid tumour of the GI tract. What is the most likely site of the primary tumour?
   a Oesophagus
   b Appendix
   c Distal ileum
   d Colon
   e Rectum

26 A patient was being investigated for colitis of unknown aetiology. Infective causes were excluded and both endoscopy and biopsy have proved inconclusive. What imaging feature would be more in keeping with ulcerative colitis than Crohn's disease?

a Fistula formation
b Evidence of ileitis
c Rectal involvement
d Skip lesions
e Stricturing

27 A patient presented with signs, symptoms and preliminary investigations suggestive of a Meckel's diverticulum. A Tc-99m pertechnetate study was positive and the patient was taken to theatre for a planned resection. At the time of surgery, no Meckel's diverticulum was identified. Other than observer error, what might explain the falsely positive Tc-99m pertechnetate study result?
a Ileal malrotation
b Intussusception
c Meckel's perforation
d Profuse gastrointestinal haemorrhage
e Rapid bowel transit

28 A 77-year-old male was investigated for chronic, intermittent low-grade gastrointestinal bleeding. He was otherwise generally well but had had an aortic valve replacement for severe aortic stenosis. Colonoscopy was unremarkable and a Tc-99m labelled red blood cell scan was performed. This showed a focus of tracer accumulation in the region of the caecum and ascending colon. During an acute episode of bleeding mesenteric angiography was performed which showed an arterial tuft and early opacification of the ileocolic vein. What is the most likely lesion to account for these appearances?
a Angiodysplasia of the colon
b Colonic carcinoma
c True arteriovenous malformation
d Colonic polyp
e Diverticular disease

29 A 44-year-old female was found to have colorectal carcinoma in the transverse colon on colonoscopy. There were no other sites of disease and no colonic polyps were seen. She remembers three immediate family members from different generations who have also been diagnosed with colonic carcinoma. As she also had occasional haematuria, imaging of her renal tract was arranged which showed a transitional cell carcinoma of the renal pelvis. Which syndrome is she most likely to have?
a Familial adenomatous polyposis
b Lynch I
c Lynch II
d Gardner's
e Turcot

30 A 66-year-old male with a small local rectal carcinoma was followed up with a restaging CT after six months' treatment. He felt generally well but had a past medical history including three previous myocardial infarctions with coronary angioplasty on two occasions. He suffered from hypercholesterolaemia and had a smoking history of 69 pack years. His exercise tolerance was poor and could only walk 50 metres before becoming breathless. No local recurrence or metastatic disease was identified but there were small bubbles of air within the lamina propria of a large proportion of the large bowel and a small amount of gas was seen in the portal vein. What is the most likely cause of the bowel abnormalities?

   a Bowel necrosis/gangrene
   b Mucosal disruption
   c Increased mucosal permeability
   d Pulmonary disease
   e Radiotherapy related

31 A premature neonate developed abdominal distension and bilious vomiting. They were being cared for in Neonatal ICU and were being treated for generalised sepsis. Necrotising enterocolitis was suspected and a plain abdominal radiograph was performed. What radiological appearance is the worst prognostic indicator?

   a Bowel dilatation
   b Free intra-abdominal air
   c Gas within the bowel wall
   d Portal vein gas
   e Thumbprinting

32 A patient previously diagnosed with HIV presented with abdominal pain, fever and malaise. Imaging findings showed a pancolitis, ascites and aphthous ulcers on a background of normal mucosa. What is the commonest cause of these findings?

   a Herpes simplex
   b *Candida*
   c *Cytomegalovirus* (CMV)
   d Tuberculosis
   e *Clostridium difficile*

33 A 37-year-old male presented with sudden onset severe abdominal pain and abdominal distension. A plain abdominal radiograph showed a distended loop of large bowel that was kidney shaped. He went on to have a contrast enhanced CT of his abdomen and pelvis. What is this most likely to show?

   a Appendicitis
   b Small bowel obstruction
   c Ischaemic bowel
   d Caecal volvulus
   e Sigmoid volvulus

34 A young patient with Crohn's disease and recurrent episodes of perianal sepsis was found to have an enterocolic fistula. What is the most likely location of this fistula?

a Ileocolic

b Ileocaecal

c Ileo-ileal

d Colo-coloic

e Ileosigmoid

35 A patient with inflammatory bowel disease was found to have colonic polyps on CT colonography. What feature would be more consistent with a diagnosis of pseudopolyposis (post-inflammatory polyposis) than true polyposis?

a Ill-defined margins

b Preserved colonic haustra

c Round

d Uniform in size

e Well-delineated

36 An elderly woman who was a long-term psychiatric inpatient was referred to the duty surgical team with symptoms of large bowel obstruction. A plain abdominal radiograph showed a grossly dilated loop of large bowel and a subsequent abdominal CT demonstrated a whirled appearance of the associated mesentery. What is the most likely diagnosis?

a Caecal volvulus

b Giant sigmoid diverticulum

c Perforated sigmoid diverticulum

d Retractile mesenteritis

e Sigmoid volvulus

37 A 37-year-old male with known alcoholic liver disease causing severe cirrhosis and multiple previous admissions for gastrointestinal haemorrhage was recently treated with a transjugular intrahepatic porto-systemic shunt (TIPS). Unfortunately, he has developed encephalopathy as a result of decompensated liver disease and the gastroenterologist would like to know if the TIPS is patent. What is the most appropriate first-line investigation to determine this?

a Ultrasound of the liver with Doppler

b Triple-phase intravenous contrast-enhanced CT

c Time of flight gadolinium-enhanced MR

d Fluoroscopy with venous catheter-based contrast injections

e Double-phase intravenous contrast-enhanced CT

38 A 35-year-old male with protein C deficiency presented with a history of a few weeks of abdominal pain, increasing abdominal distension and jaundice. Biochemistry revealed grossly abnormal liver function tests and his coagulation was also markedly abnormal. An ultrasound demonstrated widespread ascites with hypertrophy of the caudate lobe and bicoloured flow in the hepatic veins on Doppler. What is the most likely diagnosis?

   a Acute Budd-Chiari syndrome
   b Alcoholic liver disease
   c Chronic Budd-Chiari syndrome
   d Portal vein thrombosis
   e Right heart failure

39 A young woman developed haematuria and was referred for a renal tract ultrasound. She was not on any medication other than the combined oral contraceptive pill. There were no positive renal tract findings, but while scanning the right kidney the ultrasonographer noticed a solitary isoechoic lesion in the right lobe of the liver. Following further assessment, the patient was referred for a contrast-enhanced MRI, primarily to discriminate between focal nodular hyperplasia (FNH) and adenoma. What radiological finding would support a diagnosis of FNH?

   a Internal haemorrhage
   b Calcification
   c Central scar
   d Poor uptake of hepatobiliary liver contrast (Gd-BOPTA)
   e Uptake of reticuloendothelial liver contrast

40 A 42-year-old man with known alcohol-related cirrhosis was assessed in the Hepatology outpatient clinic. Blood samples were taken for serum bilirubin, albumin and prothrombin time and evidence of hepatic encephalopathy was sought clinically. An abdominal ultrasound was requested to complete Child-Pugh cirrhosis scoring. What feature of ultrasound is used to complete the Child-Pugh score?

   a Ascitic fluid
   b Collateral vessel formation
   c Portal venous flow
   d Splenomegaly
   e Varices

41 An adult patient presented with non-specific symptoms suggestive of malignancy and an abdominal ultrasound showed multiple 'target-lesions' throughout the liver consistent with hepatic metastatic deposits. Without knowing the patient's age or gender, what is the most likely site of the primary tumour?
a Breast
b Colorectal
c Bronchogenic
d Pancreatic
e Gastric

42 A gap-year student returned from a long trip to Africa having experienced a few episodes of bloody diarrhoea. She then developed increasingly severe right upper quadrant pain and was referred for an abdominal ultrasound. This showed a solitary 8-cm, hypoechoic thin-walled lesion in the right lobe of the liver. Subsequent percutaneous drainage yielded reddish brown thick fluid. What is the most likely causative organism?
a *Echinococcus* sp.
b *Entamoeba histolytica*
c *Escherichia coli*
d *Schistosoma* sp.
e *Staphylococcus aureus*

43 A 28-year-old female complained of right upper quadrant pain, dyspnoea and abdominal distension shortly after a normal vaginal delivery of her first child. Transabdominal ultrasound showed ascites and an enlarged (14 cm) spleen. What is the most likely diagnosis?
a Pulmonary embolus
b Cirrhosis
c Portal vein thrombosis
d Gastritis
e Budd-Chiari syndrome

44 A 17-year-old Greek boy presented with abdominal pain. He was of short stature but otherwise of normal physical appearance. Blood tests showed a microcytic anaemia and abnormal liver function tests. On ultrasound his liver measured 18 cm in cranio-caudal length; in the right mid-clavicular line his spleen measured 15 cm in longest axis. Gallstones were also noted in an otherwise normal gallbladder. What is the most likely diagnosis?
a Sarcoidosis
b Glycogen storage disease
c Beta-thalassaemia
d Recent viral infection
e Leukaemia

45 A young man fell 3.5 metres from a ladder and presented with severe left-sided abdominal pain. He was haemodynamically stable. Plain X-rays of the chest and abdomen were unremarkable except for multiple left-sided rib fractures. Contrast-enhanced CT of the abdomen showed a subcapsular Grade 2 splenic haematoma. How much of the spleen is likely to be involved?
a >50% of the surface area
b <25% of the surface area
c 25–50% of the surface area
d Completely shattered spleen
e <10% of the surface area

46 A middle-aged man underwent various investigations for abdominal pain and eventually was diagnosed with a splenic angiosarcoma. What signal characteristics would be expected on MRI?
a Diffuse/focal low signal on T1 and T2
b Diffuse low signal on T1, high signal T2
c Diffuse high signal on T1, low signal on T2
d Diffuse/focal high signal on T1 and T2
e Mixed foci of high and low signal on T1 and T2

47 An ultrasound in an elderly male demonstrated multiple splenic metastases. What is the most likely origin of primary?
a Colon
b Melanoma
c Prostate
d Renal cell
e Stomach

48 During an abdominal ultrasound for non-specific abdominal pain, a 52-year-old man was noted to have a focal abnormality within his spleen. A contrast-enhanced abdominal CT was then arranged which demonstrated a focal low density and minimally vascular splenic lesion and para-aortic lymphadenopathy. His serum inflammatory markers were within normal limits. What is the most likely diagnosis?
a Abscess
b Aneurysm
c Haemangioma
d Lymphoma
e Metastasis

49 A male neonate with congenital heart disease was found to have multiple spleens and a diagnosis of polysplenia syndrome was proposed. From which further abnormality is he also most likely to suffer?
a Bilateral morphological right-sided lungs
b Gut malrotation
c Hepatic fibrosis

d Imperforate anus

e Undescended testes

50 An overweight elderly female patient with a strong smoking history had an ultrasound of her abdomen and pelvis. Her gallbladder contained some small stones and the wall measured 2-mm thick except for an irregular focal area that was 6-mm thick. There was no acoustic shadowing from this thickened area. The gallbladder was of normal volume and the bile ducts were not dilated. What is the most likely diagnosis?

a Carcinoma of the gallbladder

b Hyperplastic cholecystoses

c Inflammatory polyp

d Metastases from malignant melanoma

e Wall-adherent gallstone

51 A middle-aged male underwent an ultrasound of his abdomen which showed sludge within a thin-walled gallbladder and no calculi. How likely is it that this patient will go on to develop gallstones?

a 0%

b 5–15%

c 30–45%

d 60–70%

e 95%

52 An elderly gentleman was admitted with severe abdominal pain, jaundice and sepsis. He had a significant cardiac history, suffered from chronic airways disease and was a high anaesthetic risk. An ultrasound and CT confirmed severe calculus cholecystitis with a distended gallbladder but no common bile duct dilation. The patient was not responding well to intravenous antibiotic therapy and continued to deteriorate. What would be the most appropriate next step?

a ERCP

b Laparoscopic cholecystectomy

c MRCP

d Open cholecystectomy

e Percutaneous cholecystostomy

53 A 75-year-old female had an abdominal radiograph as part of a work-up for chronic right upper quadrant pain. This showed a porcelain gallbladder. She subsequently has a transabdominal ultrasound which showed a fundal mass in the gallbladder, but no gallstones and gallbladder carcinoma was suspected. What is the most common mode of spread?

a Infiltration of liver

b Neural spread

c Lymphatic spread to cystic nodes

d Lymphatic spread to coeliac nodes

e Haematogenous

54 A 20-year-old woman presented with ongoing chronic vague abdominal pain. She was otherwise well and was taking the oral contraceptive pill. On examination there was a palpable mass in the right upper quadrant and her sclera appeared yellow. An urgent outpatient ultrasound was organised and a choledochocele was suspected. What ultrasound finding would support this diagnosis?

a Cystic change of the intrahepatic ducts

b Dilatation of the distal intramural portion of the common bile duct that protrudes in the duodenum

c Diverticular outpouching of the extrahepatic duct

d Fusiform dilatation of the extrahepatic duct

e Multifocal saccular dilatation of the intraheptic ducts with sparing of the extrahepatic ducts

55 A patient presented with right upper quadrant pain, fever and jaundice. An ultrasound demonstrated a thick-walled gallbladder containing numerous gallstones and a stone impacted in the common bile duct. Which organism is most likely to be grown from their blood cultures?

a *Pseudomonas*

b *Klebsiella*

c *Escherichia coli*

d *Haemophilus influenzae*

e *Clostridium difficile*

56 Following a long history of intermittent right upper quadrant pain a middle-aged woman became jaundiced. She was referred for an ultrasound which showed a cystic lesion adjacent to the gallbladder. A CT confirmed the presence of a thin-walled lesion with a fluid attenuation centre. The intrahepatic ducts were normal in calibre. In view of her jaundice she then had an ERCP and a cholangiogram showed a tubular structure which communicated with the gallbladder and cystic duct. What is the most likely diagnosis?

a Biloma

b Caroli's disease

c Choledochal cyst

d Enteric duplication cyst

e Pancreatic pseudocyst

57 A 23-year-old male presented with his third episode of right upper quadrant pain, fever and jaundice in six months. A contrast-enhanced CT showed multiple intrahepatic cysts, some of which showed strongly enhancing tiny central dots and focal calcification. There were also cystic foci in the renal parenchyma bilaterally. What is the most likely diagnosis?

a Polycystic liver disease

b Biliary haemangioma

c Primary sclerosing cholangitis

    d Caroli's disease

    e Ascending cholangitis

58 A 55-year-old man presented with painless jaundice and was diagnosed with extrahepatic cholangiocarcinoma. What is the most common mode of spread?

    a Infiltration of liver

    b Peritoneal seeding

    c Lymphatic spread to cystic lymph nodes

    d Lymphatic spread to coeliac lymph nodes

    e Haematogenous

59 A 40-year-old woman presented with right upper quadrant pain. A transabdominal ultrasound showed multiple gallstones in a thick-walled gallbladder with a trace of pericholecystic free fluid. She subsequently developed a biliary enteric fistula. What is the most likely site of communication with the gastrointestinal tract?

    a Duodenum

    b Colon

    c Stomach

    d Jejunum

    e Ileum

60 A previously well 40-year-old woman was admitted with a one-week history of right upper quadrant pain and vomiting. An abdominal radiograph taken on admission showed dilated small bowel loops containing a number of lamellated calcific densities and pneumobilia. What is the most likely diagnosis?

    a Acute cholecystitis

    b Acute pancreatitis

    c Cholangitis

    d Gallstone ileus

    e Gastric volvulus

61 A 30-year-old female smoker was investigated for general malaise and epigastric discomfort with a transabdominal ultrasound. This showed gallstones in a thin-walled gallbladder and echogenic soft tissue around the distal common bile duct and pancreatic head but no dilatation of any of the duct system. What is the most likely diagnosis?

    a Pancreatic head carcinoma

    b Chronic pancreatitis

    c Impacted distal CBD stone

    d Lymphoma

    e Pancreatic metastasis

62 A 46-year-old male presented with a one-year history of vague epigastric pain. He had a history of ischaemic heart disease and hypercholesterolaemia. On examination there was mild hepatomegaly. Inflammatory markers, amylase and liver function tests were within normal limits. An abdominal ultrasound showed multiple hyperechoic focal deposits in the liver but obscuration of central structures by bowel gas. A CT was performed which showed two small (1-cm) lesions within the body of the pancreas that enhanced avidly in arterial phase. The liver lesions were also hypervascular. What is the most likely diagnosis?

a Hepatocellular carcinoma
b Lymphoma
c Pancreatic acinar cell carcinoma
d Pancreatic ductal adenocarcinoma
e Pancreatic islet cell tumour

63 A patient who was spiking temperatures on their fifth post-operative day underwent an abdominal CT. This showed reordered anatomy with a gastrojejunostomy, choledochojejunostomy and pancreaticojejunostomy. There was a small amount of free fluid and free air and more marked pneumobilia. What surgical procedure has been performed?

a Roux-en-Y choledochojejunostomy
b Roux-en-Y with post-operative complications
c Roux-en-Y normal with normal post-operative appearances
d Whipple's procedure with post-operative complications
e Whipple's procedure with normal post-operative appearances

64 A 16-year-old boy was involved in a road traffic accident and a multi-trauma CT was performed. He had a history of several previous admissions for acute abdominal pain that had remained undiagnosed and his father had died aged 36 of pancreatic carcinoma. The CT showed a sterna fracture, lung contusions and a femoral fracture. Additionally, there were several large spherical calcifications within the pancreas and a 4-cm pseudocyst with relative preservation of the gland volume. He made a good recovery from his acute injuries but follow-up was considered for his pancreatic findings. What is the most likely diagnosis?

a Cystic fibrosis
b Hereditary pancreatitis
c Pancreas divisum
d Post-mumps pancreatitis
e Trauma

65 A patient on the ITU was recovering from multi-organ failure after a severe episode of acute pancreatitis when his haemoglobin dropped by 3 g/dL over two days. Intra-abdominal haemorrhage was suspected and CT angiography demonstrated a contrast blush adjacent to an apparently aneurysmal vessel very near the pancreas itself. Which vessel is most likely to be involved?

a Gastroduodenal artery
b Inferior pancreaticoduodenal artery
c Pancreatic arcade arteries
d Splenic artery
e Superior pancreaticoduodenal artery

66 A 44-year-old obese lady was admitted with an episode of acute pancreatitis. Blood tests showed abnormal liver function and a leucocytosis. Her renal function was normal and no complication was clinically evident. Which investigation is most appropriate in this situation?
a Contrast-enhanced CT abdomen and pelvis in 7–10 days
b Immediate contrast enhanced CT abdomen and pelvis
c Immediate contrast-enhanced CT chest, abdomen and pelvis
d No imaging required at present
e Ultrasound of the abdomen

67 A young boy presented after hitting the handlebars of his push bike. Imaging demonstrated pancreatic parenchymal damage that did not involve the main pancreatic duct. What grade of injury has he suffered?
a Grade I injury
b Grade II injury
c Grade III injury
d Grade IV injury
e Grade V injury

68 During abdominal ultrasound a patient was noted to have an echogenic pancreas with areas of hypoechogenicity. A contrast-enhanced CT scan was subsequently performed which showed multiple pancreatic cysts. There was no lymphadenopathy. What further feature would make a mucinous cystic neoplasm more likely?
a Cysts with near fluid density
b Calcification
c Hypovascularity
d Cysts of 20 mm in size
e Patient in their eighth decade

69 An otherwise fit 54-year-old man presented with non-specific abdominal pain and weight loss. An ultrasound and subsequent CT with biopsy confirmed a diagnosis of pancreatic adenocarcinoma. A resection was planned and the CT was reviewed. Which of the following features is most compatible with a resectable tumour?
a Dilatation of pancreatic duct
b Direct tumour extension of tumour into left hepatic lobe
c Encasement of the superior mesenteric artery
d Thickening of Gerota's fascia
e 2-cm regional lymph node

70 A 34-year-old Indian male was assessed in the Gastroenterology outpatient clinic with a one-year history of weight loss and vague abdominal discomfort. His chest radiograph was of normal appearance and his tuberculin skin test was negative, but he had multiple risk factors for tuberculous disease. Primary intestinal tuberculosis was considered as a possibility and barium studies of the small bowel were arranged which showed disease in the ilea-caecal area. What characteristic would most support tuberculosis as a diagnosis?

a Cobblestoning
b Deep fissures and large shallow linear ulcers with elevated margins
c Longitudinal submucosal ulceration over several centimetres
d Presence of multiple ulcers that resemble 'rose thorns'
e Presence of pseudopolyps

Gastrointestinal and hepatobiliary radiology

PAPER 3

1   A 55-year-old male with a history of drug and alcohol abuse underwent an elective barium swallow for follow-up after surgery for laryngeal carcinoma. This demonstrated tortuous longitudinal filling defects in the lower third of a partially collapsed oesophagus. What is the most likely cause of these radiological findings?
    a   Oesophageal varices
    b   Mucosal oedema associated with oesophagitis
    c   Oesophageal lymphoma
    d   Varicoid oesophageal carcinoma
    e   Achalasia

2   A patient attending for an abdominal ultrasound scan was noted to have a focal abnormality within the liver, which lies high within the right lobe and abuts the right hepatic vein. Which segment is the lesion most likely to involve?
    a   4A
    b   4B
    c   5
    d   6
    e   7

3   A 33-year-old woman presented with abdominal pain and distension. A plain abdominal radiograph showed small bowel obstruction and a CT was performed which showed a transition point in a segment of small bowel. What feature would suggest that this is jejunal as opposed to an ileal segment?
    a   Sparse/absent valvulae conniventes
    b   More frequent arterial arcades
    c   Thicker valvulae conniventes
    d   Thinner bowel wall
    e   Slightly smaller diameter than rest of small bowel

4 A 44-year-old female underwent an elective barium swallow to investigate a long history of reflux oesophagitis, which was poorly controlled with proton pump inhibitors. The report concluded that an inflammatory oesophagogastric polyp was identified, which was confirmed on endoscopy. What descriptive findings would be most likely to support this conclusion?
   a Large pedunculated mass with sausage-shaped appearance
   b Plaque-like, sessile polyp
   c Polypoid protuberance arising near cardia
   d Sessile, slightly lobulated polyp
   e Smooth submucosal mass in distal third of oesophagus

5 A patient from South America had an elective barium swallow to investigate weight loss. This showed diffuse oesophageal dilation. He has a history of cardiomyopathy and megacolon. What is the most likely diagnosis?
   a Amyloidosis
   b Chagas disease
   c Oesophagitis
   d Scleroderma
   e Systemic lupus erythematosus

6 A 35-year-old male presented with weight loss and dysphagia to both solids and liquids. A plain CXR and AXR were unremarkable and a contrast swallow showed a mildly dilated oesophagus with absent primary and secondary peristaltic waves. Tertiary contractions were seen and the lower oesophagus had a beak-like appearance. What is the most likely pathology?
   a Achalasia
   b Adenocarcinoma
   c Presbyesophagus
   d Oesophageal spasm
   e Scleroderma

7 A middle-aged male had a barium swallow to investigate dysphagia. This showed a smooth, lobulated, well-defined lesion that was subsequently found to be intramural. What is the most likely cause of this appearance?
   a Oesophageal polyp
   b Squamous cell carcinoma
   c Presbyesophagus
   d Oesophageal leiomyoma
   e Hiatus hernia

8 A patient, who was known to be HIV positive, underwent a contrast swallow to investigate painful swallowing. A large oesophageal ulcer with a well-defined rim was demonstrated. The oesophageal mucosa was otherwise normal and there were no strictures or motility anomalies. What is the most likely diagnosis?
   a Barrett's oesophagus
   b CMV oesophagitis

c Drug-induced oesophagitis
d Malignant ulceration
e Radiation oesophagitis

9   A previously fit and well 36-year-old man developed dysphagia to solid food
    and was referred for a contrast swallow. The reporting radiologist noticed large
    volume mediastinal lymphadenopathy and following contrast a large, poly-
    poidal oesophageal mass was visible. What is the most likely diagnosis?
    a Oesophageal carcinoma
    b Lymphoma
    c Oesophageal haematoma
    d Submucosal metastases
    e Oesophageal varices

10 A 92-year-old woman presented with repeated episodes of aspiration pneu-
    monia. A contrast swallow showed an oesophageal diverticulum. What
    feature would make a Zenker's diverticulum more likely than an alternative
    diagnosis?
    a Anterior position
    b Multiple diverticula
    c Origin below cricopharyngeus
    d Origin at Killian's dehiscence
    e Static appearance of diverticulum during swallow

11 A 54-year-old man with histologically confirmed adenocarcinoma at the
    gastro-oesophageal junction underwent FDG PET-CT for further staging.
    This demonstrated significant uptake (>2.5 SUV) at the site of the tumour,
    an adjacent local nodal mass and gastro-hepatic and coeliac axis nodes. No
    other abnormal uptake was seen in the chest, abdomen or pelvis. What is the
    most appropriate staging for this patient?
    a N1 M1b
    b N2 M0
    c N1 M1a
    d N1 M1b
    e N1 Mx

12 A patient presented three weeks after a laparoscopic cholecystectomy with
    increasing abdominal pain and raised inflammatory markers. An ultrasound
    showed an ill-defined low-reflectivity mass adjacent to the inferior surface
    of the liver with no increased Doppler signal. What is the best investigation
    to establish if the mass is a biloma?
    a Triple-phase contrast-enhanced CT of the abdomen and pelvis
    b Magnetic resonance cholangiopancreatography (MRCP)
    c Radionuclide HIDA scan
    d White cell labelled Tc scan
    e Radionuclide bile salt malabsorption study

13 A neonate presented with bile-stained vomiting, which started after its first feed. A plain abdominal radiograph showed a 'double bubble'. The child also had an umbilical hernia, Brushfield spots and a single palmar crease. What is the most likely diagnosis?

a Annular pancreas
b Duodenal atresia
c Duodenal stenosis
d Ladd bands
e Pyloric stenosis

14 A 37-year-old male presented with gastric outlet obstruction. He had a history of epigastric pain related to food and an abdominal CT showed a dilated stomach with irregular inflammatory narrowing in the distal stomach. What is the most likely cause?

a Antral carcinoma
b Crohn's disease
c Peptic ulcer disease
d Sarcoidosis
e Syphilis

15 A 55-year-old male presented with severe symptoms of reflux. A barium study showed thickened gastric rugae, duodenal and jejunal folds and multiple peptic ulcers. His serum gastrin level was elevated. What is the most likely diagnosis?

a Barrett's oesophagus
b Oesophageal Crohn's disease
c Zollinger-Ellison syndrome
d Pancreatitis
e Helicobacter pylori infection

16 A patient presented three months after a gastrojejunostomy with left to right anastomosis with epigastric fullness relieved by bilious vomiting, and B12 deficiency. CT demonstrated a fluid dense mass adjacent to the head of the pancreas with a further similar mass near the tail of the pancreas. What diagnosis are these findings most suggestive of?

a Anastomotic leak
b Blind loop syndrome
c Incorrect anastomosis
d Anastomotic dehiscence
e Gastric volvulus

17 A 50-year-old landscape gardener presented with abdominal pain and was assessed with a CT scan on which gastric mucosal irregularity was noted. His pain settled with conservative management and he was followed up with a barium meal as an outpatient, which showed multiple target ('bull's-eye') lesions in the stomach.
a Pancreatic 'rest'
b Gastric Crohn's disease
c Gastric carcinoma
d Neurofibroma
e Submucosal metastases

18 A patient was noted to have an abnormal appearance of the stomach wall on abdominal CT. A barium meal was subsequently performed and a diagnosis of ectopic pancreatic tissue (pancreatic rest) was considered. What finding would be most typical of this diagnosis?
a Dots and linear streaks of barium
b Featureless gastric mucosa
c Multiple aphthous ulcers
d Polypoid fundal mass
e Submucosal umbilicated mass

19 Following an episode of haematemesis a 48-year-old man visited his doctor. He admitted several months of dyspeptic symptoms, some weight loss and said he had been drinking up to a bottle of spirit daily. He was referred for an endoscopy, which he was not able to tolerate. Consequently, a barium meal was performed which showed a large ulcer within an oedematous mound on the greater curvature. What further feature would suggest a malignant ulcer?
a Carman's (meniscus) sign
b Central location of ulcer within mound
c Extension of mucosal folds to crater edge
d Hampton's line
e Thin mucosal folds

20 A 31-year-old man was involved in a high-speed road accident and sustained significant chest and head injuries. He was admitted to ITU and a chest radiograph obtained 24 hours later showed pneumoperitoneum. An occult gut injury was suspected. What part of the gut is most likely to have been injured?
a Gastro-oesophageal junction
b Duodenum
c Ileum
d Colon
e Rectum

21 A 55-year-old male who was previously well, presented with a short history of per rectum bleeding and weight loss. Physical examination was normal and a colonoscopy was not available. A contrast-enhanced CT was performed which showed a submucosal vascular lesion in the ileum with associated moderate-volume low-density lymphadenopathy. In addition, in the sigmoid colon, there was an area of irregular but concentric wall thickening consistent with a colonic carcinoma. What is the likely aetiology of each abnormality?

   a Colorectal primary carcinoma with small bowel metastases and lymph node involvement
   b Carcinoid of the small bowel with large bowel metastases
   c Small bowel carcinoma with large bowel metastases
   d Concurrent colorectal and small bowel primary carcinoma
   e Carcinoid of small bowel with a concurrent colorectal malignancy

22 A 39-year-old male presented with abdominal pain, vomiting and a distended abdomen. A plain abdominal radiograph showed dilated loops of small bowel. He was otherwise well with no previous surgery and his hernial orifices were normal. A contrast-enhanced CT showed an internal encapsulated bowel loop, which was displacing the inferior mesenteric vein. What is the most likely cause for these appearances?

   a Right paraduodenal hernia
   b Left paraduodenal hernia
   c Lesser sac hernia
   d Intersigmoid hernia
   e Inguinal hernia

23 A patient presents for review following a CT of their abdomen and pelvis in another centre. The images have not been transferred but the report describes an enhancing submucosal mass in the ileum with associated changes in the mesentery. The report continues describing a stellate radiating pattern and beading of the mesenteric neurovascular bundles with retraction of the mesentery and thickening of the wall of the subtended loops of bowel. Assuming the report is accurate, what is the most likely diagnosis?

   a Lymphoma
   b Metastatic gastric carcinoma
   c Carcinoid tumour
   d Mesenteric panniculitis
   e Gardner's syndrome

24 An 18-year-old girl presented with a one-year history of recurrent colicky abdominal pain, diarrhoea, anorexia and weight loss. Blood tests showed an iron deficiency anaemia. Gastroscopy and colonoscopy as far as the hepatic flexure were normal. A small bowel follow-through showed thickened ileal folds, aphthous ulcers, cobblestoning and terminal ileal stricturing. What is the most likely diagnosis?

   a Crohn's disease

b Ulcerative colitis

c Bowel ischaemia

d Appendicitis

e Mesenteric venous thrombosis

25 A 28-year-old male presented with abdominal pain and diarrhoea. A CT demonstrated an oedematous terminal ileum with large penetrating ulcers. Further clinical examination revealed stomatitis, genital ulcers and iridocyclitis. What is the most likely diagnosis?

a Ulcerative colitis

b Crohn's disease

c Behcet's syndrome

d Mirizzi's syndrome

e Herpes simplex infection

26 A 65-year-old woman was investigated for recurrent diarrhoea. Her husband reported that she also became flushed and slightly short of breath after meals. Carcinoid syndrome was suspected and she was referred for an abdominal CT and small bowel MRI study. What feature is most typical of small bowel carcinoid?

a Duodenal location

b Calcified lymphadenopathy

c Mesenteric mass

d Minimal desmoplastic reaction

e Free fluid

27 A 20-year-old woman developed an urticarial rash, flushing, diarrhoea and abdominal discomfort. An abdominal CT demonstrated irregular small bowel fold thickening and a subsequent small bowel contrast study showed multiple tiny small bowel nodules. What is the most likely diagnosis?

a Amyloidosis

b Coeliac disease

c Nodular lymphoid hyperplasia

d Small bowel carcinoid

e Systemic mastocytosis

28 A 32-year-old female was diagnosed with Crohn's disease. She had ongoing problems with recto-anal fistulae and was keen to explore a surgical solution if appropriate. The last CT of her abdomen and pelvis was performed over 18 months ago and the inflammation is currently relatively quiescent. What is the most appropriate way of further investigating the fistulae?

a MR fistulography

b Contrast enema

c Transrectal ultrasound

d No imaging, surgical exploration only

e Repeat contrast-enhanced CT

29 An elderly patient with acute lower gastrointestinal bleeding underwent mesenteric angiography with the aim of identifying and treating the source of the bleeding. Which is the usual order to performing this study?

   a The superior mesenteric artery is evaluated before the inferior mesenteric artery

   b The inferior mesenteric artery is evaluated before the superior mesenteric artery

   c There is no recommended order; evaluation should be based on the order in which the arteries happen to be catheterised

   d The coeliac axis is evaluated before the superior mesenteric artery

   e The renal arteries are evaluated first, followed by the other vessels in any order

30 A 58-year-old male with rectal carcinoma underwent staging with CT and MRI. The MRI reported 'there is transmural extension of the local disease but no invasion of adjacent organs. There is a single lymph node measuring 1.2 cm in the short axis seen within the mesorectal envelope'. No distant disease was seen on the CT. On the basis of this information what is the TMN staging?

   a T2 N0 M0

   b T2 N1 M0

   c T3 N0 M0

   d T3 N1 M0

   e T4 N1 M0

31 A 65-year-old male presented with severe acute abdominal pain. He had a past history of ischaemic heart disease and was in atrial fibrillation. He had diffuse abdominal pain with generalised tenderness but was not peritonitic. Blood tests showed raised inflammatory markers and blood gases demonstrated a metabolic acidosis with a raised lactate. A plain abdominal radiograph showed thumbprinting of the colon wall and a contrast-enhanced CT demonstrated colonic mucosal oedema, sparing the small bowel and rectum. What is the most likely diagnosis?

   a Crohn's disease

   b Ulcerative colitis

   c Ischaemic colitis

   d Sigmoid volvulus

   e Pancreatitis

32 A 58-year-old male presented with intermittent low-grade rectal bleeding. Angiography showed a cluster of vessels on the anti-mesenteric border in the caecal region in arterial phase with early opacification of an ileo-colic vein and a densely opacified tortuous ileo-colic vein in the late venous phase. What is the most likely diagnosis?

   a Meckel's diverticulum

   b Angiodysplasia

c Crohn's disease
d Caecal ulcer
e Caecal carcinoma

33 An elderly depressed patient was admitted from his nursing home on numerous occasions with abdominal pain and distension. On each occasion a plain abdominal radiograph was performed which showed multiple distended fluid-filled loops of bowel with the appearance of a 'coffee bean'. What is the most likely diagnosis?
a Appendicitis
b Small bowel obstruction
c Ischaemic bowel
d Caecal volvulus
e Sigmoid volvulus

34 A patient underwent a barium enema as an investigation for change in bowel habit. Apart from a few diverticula the only positive finding was widening of the pre-sacral space. In 95% of cases, what is the accepted value for a normal pre-sacral space?
a >5 mm
b <5 mm
c >10 mm
d 15 mm
e >15 mm

35 An 80-year-old female presented with a history of passing blood and mucus per rectum. She had no history of weight loss or inflammatory bowel disease and no family history of colorectal cancer. She was unable to tolerate bowel preparation and was therefore referred for a minimally prepared CT colon. A polyp was visible in her descending colon. What further finding would most suggest this polyp was malignant?
a 1.5 cm in size
b Lobulation
c Pedunculated
d Solitary
e Smooth underlying colonic wall

36 A young HIV-positive man presented with localised peritonism and was further assessed with CT. He had recently had a positive stool culture for *Salmonella*, which was felt to be responsible for his symptoms. Which part of the bowel is most likely to appear abnormal on CT?
a Terminal ileum
b Right hemicolon
c Left hemicolon
d Sigmoid
e Entire colon

37 A middle-aged female underwent an abdominal ultrasound which demonstrated an area of increased reflectivity within the right lobe of her liver. She has no significant past medical history and a benign haemangioma is suspected. Were she to have an MRI what would the most likely signal characteristics of this lesion be?

a Hypointense T1 and hyperintense T2

b Hypointense T1 and hypointense T2

c Hyperintense T1 and hyperintense T2

d Hyperintense T1 and hypointense T2

e Hyperintense T1 and isointense T2

38 A patient with shortness of breath underwent abdominal ultrasound which showed a thick-walled gallbladder but no gallstones. They were pain free and routine serum biochemical markers including C-reactive protein, albumin, eGFR and liver transaminases were normal. What is the most likely explanation for the gallbladder wall thickening?

a Cirrhosis

b Viral hepatitis

c Cardiac failure

d Renal failure

e Cholecystitis

39 Which of the following is an expected normal finding following liver transplant?

a Hepatic arterial resistive index <0.5

b Hepatic infarction

c Increased periportal attenuation

d Periportal lymphadenopathy

e Portal vein thrombosis

40 A focal liver abnormality was detected in a middle-aged man and he subsequently underwent a liver MRI to further delineate the lesion. The MRI showed the lesion to be hyperintense on T1-weighted sequences and hypointense on T2-weighted sequences. What lesion is most likely to exhibit this pattern of signal return?

a Adenoma

b Regenerative nodule

c Focal nodular hyperplasia

d Haemangioma

e Metastases

41 A patient with a known colorectal carcinoma was being investigated for possible liver metastases. What modality is most sensitive in detecting liver metastases?
    a Contrast-enhanced CT
    b ERCP
    c MRI
    d FDG PET-CT
    e Ultrasound

42 A middle-aged man, known to have acute leukaemia, was referred for an abdominal ultrasound. Several small, uniformly hypoechoic nodules were visible within the liver, which were thought to represent foci of hepatic candidiasis and resolved following empirical treatment with antifungal drugs. Via what route is it most likely that the fungal infection spread to the liver?
    a Biliary ducts
    b Hepatic artery
    c Percutaneous
    d Portal vein
    e Transcoelomic

43 A 30-year-old man with known polycythaemia rubra vera was referred for contrast-enhanced CT for investigation of progressive abdominal distension and jaundice. This showed ascites, caudate and right hepatic lobar hypertrophy with mosaic enhancement of the liver. There was also a low attenuation 2-cm lesion in segment 2 which showed peripheral nodular enhancement. A delayed phase scan showed filling in of the segment 2 lesion, but the remaining liver enhancement was markedly delayed. What is the most likely diagnosis?
    a Hepatocellular carcinoma
    b Liver metastases
    c Cirrhotic liver disease
    d Budd-Chiari syndrome
    e Alcoholic hepatitis

44 A 78-year-old female presented with left upper quadrant pain and a fever. Her past medical history included multiple myocardial infarctions, subsequent coronary artery bypass surgery, non-insulin dependent diabetes and poorly controlled hypertension. Initial baseline blood tests were unremarkable except for a mild leucocytosis. An ultrasound of her abdomen demonstrated a single ill-defined wedge-shaped area of decreased reflectivity within the spleen. What is the most likely diagnosis?
    a Primary splenic malignancy
    b Secondary splenic malignancy
    c Splenic infarct secondary to embolic phenomenon
    d Splenic infarct secondary to local thrombus
    e Splenic abscess

45 In a normal unenhanced CT scan of the upper abdomen, the liver parenchyma measures 65 HU. What would be the expected density of the spleen?
 a 20–30 HU
 b 40–60 HU
 c 65 HU
 d 70–80 HU
 e 100–120 HU

46 A patient underwent a CT of the upper abdomen as part of a lung cancer staging scan. This demonstrated multiple wedge-shaped peripheral lesions of low attenuation within the spleen in both the arterial and portal venous phases. This was not thought to be due to metastases from the lung cancer. What is the commonest cause of this appearance?
 a Atheroma
 b Bacterial endocarditis
 c Non-Hodgkin's lymphoma
 d Polycythaemia rubra vera
 e Sickle cell disease

47 A plain abdominal radiograph was performed on a patient with suspected bowel obstruction. This was unremarkable apart from multiple well-defined calcifications that were diffusely distributed throughout the region of the spleen. What is the most likely cause of this appearance?
 a Epidermoid cysts
 b Granulomas
 c Haematomas
 d Phleboliths
 e Splenic artery aneurysms

48 A 37-year-old Afro-Caribbean woman with suspected erythema nodosum was referred to a dermatologist. On physical examination she was noted to have a palpable spleen and an abdominal ultrasound was requested. This demonstrated moderate splenic enlargement and scattered nodular lesions throughout the liver and spleen. What it the most likely unifying diagnosis?
 a Amyloidosis
 b Chronic myeloid leukaemia
 c Malaria
 d Sarcoidosis
 e Untreated lymphoma

49 A diabetic 70-year-old man was admitted with right upper quadrant pain. He became rapidly more unwell with evidence of sepsis and an urgent ultrasound of his abdomen was arranged. A previous ultrasound six months ago demonstrated stones within the gallbladder but little else. What feature on the more recent scan would suggest a diagnosis of the more unusual emphysematous cholecystitis over simple acute cholecystitis?

a Arc-like hyperechogenic areas outlining the gallbladder wall
b Gallbladder wall thickening over 5 mm
c Hazy delineation of the gallbladder
d Intramural gas
e The 'halo sign'

50 A US abdomen of a 37-year-old lady with a one-month history of intermittent right upper quadrant pain showed an abnormality within the gallbladder. There was no further abnormality elsewhere. What feature on ultrasound would be more in keeping with sludge rather than a polyp?
a Hyper-reflective
b Non-shadowing and mobile
c Non-shadowing and non-mobile
d Shadowing and mobile
e Shadowing and non-mobile

51 A patient underwent an abdominal ultrasound on which it was difficult to identify her gallbladder but there was a large amount of pericholecystic fluid. The patient then had a contrast-enhanced CT which demonstrated pockets of air in the gallbladder wall and abnormal mucosal enhancement of the gallbladder wall with a small defect laterally. What is the most likely diagnosis?
a Acute acalculous cholecystitis
b Acute calculus cholecystitis
c Emphysematous cholecystitis
d Gangrenous cholecystitis
e Gallbladder perforation

52 A 50-year-old man with type 2 diabetes was diagnosed with acute cholecystitis. Transabdominal ultrasound showed gas artefact echoes outlining the gallbladder wall. What is the most likely causative organism?
a *Clostridium difficile*
b *Clostridium perfringens*
c *Escherichia coli*
d *Staphylococcus aureus*
e *Staphylococcus epidermidis*

53 A 40-year-old woman was admitted with colicky right upper quadrant pain. An ultrasound showed a thick-walled gallbladder but no gallstones. Subsequently, scintigraphy was performed to assess the patency of her cystic duct. What is the most specific sign of an impacted cystic duct stone?
a Non-visualisation of the gallbladder by one hour
b Non-visualisation of the gallbladder by four hours
c Non-visualisation of the GB and CBD
d Pericholecystic rim sign
e Increased perfusion to gallbladder fossa during arterial phase

54 A 55-year-old male had been complaining of general malaise and weight loss for approximately six months. He had a past medical history of a total colectomy in early adulthood following a diagnosis of a familial adenomatous polyposis syndrome. CT and MRCP demonstrated double duct dilation. No other pathology was identified and an endoscopy was also unremarkable. What is the most likely diagnosis?

a Ampullary stricture
b Ampullary tumour
c Choledochocele
d Gallstone impaction at the ampulla
e Peri-ampullary tumour

55 A 45-year-old man presented with progressive jaundice and abnormal liver function tests. An ultrasound of his liver showed bright portal tracts and a filling defect in the common bile duct. An ERCP demonstrated multifocal strictures particularly at the bifurcations of the biliary ducts and a 'string of beads' appearance. Small saccular outpouchings were also visible. What is the most likely diagnosis?

a Primary sclerosing cholangitis
b Cholangiocarcinoma
c Bacterial cholangitis
d Primary biliary cirrhosis
e Gallbladder perforation

56 A patient with known cholelithiasis developed jaundice and underwent ultrasound and subsequent MRCP which confirmed a diagnosis of Mirizzi's syndrome. What radiological features would be expected?

a Course of cystic duct perpendicular to common hepatic duct
b Dilatation of common bile duct to the ampulla
c Impacted gallstone in the pouch of Douglas
d Air in the intrahepatic ducts
e Fistulation between the gallbladder and common hepatic duct

57 A 36-year-old woman who was known to be HIV positive presented with right upper quadrant pain, jaundice and a fever. An admission USS liver showed dilated thick-walled bile ducts. She was diagnosed with an opportunistic infection. What is the most likely causative organism?

a *Pneumocystis (PCP)*
b *Cryptococcus*
c HIV
d *Cytomegalovirus*
e *Escherichia coli*

58 A 55-year-old man presented with a three-month history of right upper quadrant pain and two-stone weight loss. On examination there was a tender palpable mass. His serum bilirubin was 15 micromoll/L and his alkaline phosphatase 200 IU/L. An ultrasound showed a hyperechoic 5-cm mass in the lateral right lobe of the liver and dilated bile ducts peripheral to this area. A CT showed this mass to be hypodense and early rim enhancement followed by marked homogeneous delayed enhancement was visible. What is the most likely diagnosis?

  a Metastatic adenocarcinoma
  b Metastatic leiomyosarcoma
  c Intrahepatic cholangiocarcinoma
  d Hepatocellular carcinoma
  e Carcinoid

59 An 18-year-old woman was investigated for right upper quadrant pain and two episodes of jaundice. An ultrasound showed a large cyst below the porta hepatis, which was separate from gallbladder and communicated with the common hepatic duct. A HIDA scan showed only equivocal uptake. What is the most likely diagnosis?

  a Hepatic cyst
  b Intrahepatic gallbladder
  c Pancreatic pseudocyst
  d Biloma
  e Choledochal cyst

60 A 55-year-old man had been diagnosed with ulcerative colitis aged 40 and had a total colectomy at 42 years old. He had been asymptomatic until presenting with a one-month history of right upper quadrant pain and jaundice. Transabdominal ultrasound showed prominent right intrahepatic ducts with echogenic walls. What is the most likely diagnosis?

  a Portal vein thrombosis
  b Primary biliary cirrhosis
  c Intrahepatic cholangiocarcinoma
  d Ascending cholangitis
  e Viral hepatis

61 A one-month-old baby girl with a persistent productive cough developed progressively worsening respiratory distress. She had a chest radiograph which showed clear lungs. Linear gas shadows were visible projected over the central liver. What is the most likely diagnosis?

  a Respiratory distress syndrome
  b Bronchopneumonia
  c Tracheoesophageal fistula
  d Congenital tracheobiliary fistula
  e Pulmonary emboli

62 A 38-year-old male with a history of alcohol and drug abuse attended the Emergency Department with severe abdominal pain. His amylase was 5105 IU/L and a diagnosis of pancreatitis was made. The patient was resuscitated and transferred to the surgical ward where, after four days, he became more unwell. A CT was then performed which showed gland oedema, inflammatory changes in the surrounding retroperitoneal fat and hyperdense areas (50–70 HU) within the gland. What is the most likely diagnosis?
a Haemorrhagic pancreatitis
b Pancreatic calcification
c Pancreatic necrosis
d Phlegmonous pancreatitis
e Suppurative pancreatitis

63 A young female was admitted with generalised lower abdominal pain. She had a mild pyrexia and borderline raised inflammatory markers. Appendicitis was considered as a diagnosis and an ultrasound was requested. What ultrasound finding would be most supportive of this?
a Compressible tubular structure >4 mm thick
b Non-compressible tubular structure >4 mm thick
c Compressible tubular structure >6 mm thick
d Non-compressible tubular structure >6 mm thick
e Wall thickness of 1 mm

64 An obese 40-year-old male who had been diagnosed with MEN type 1 via genetic screening underwent an abdominal MRI. Two lesions measuring 2.5 and 2 cm were identified in the pancreas. They were hypointense on T1- and hyperintense on T2-weighted images and there was ring enhancement after gadolinium administration. What is the most likely pancreatic pathology?
a Glucagonoma
b Gastrinoma
c Insulinoma
d Non-functioning islet cell tumour
e VIPoma

65 An eight-year-old boy was admitted after falling onto the handle bars of his bike and then onto the road. In addition to significant musculoskeletal injuries he complained of abdominal pain and on examination had a rigid abdomen with minimal bowel sounds. An ultrasound of the abdomen showed a small amount of intra-abdominal free fluid and as he was becoming more unwell an urgent CT was performed. This showed oedema in the peri-pancreatic fat and irregularity of the pancreatic contour. A discrete ill-defined area of low attenuation was seen in the region of the junction of the body and tail and there was bilateral thickening of the para-renal fascia. There was no appreciable loss of gland volume and pancreatic duct was normal. What is the most likely conclusion on the basis of these imaging findings?

a Major ductal injury
b Major vascular injury
c Pancreatic contusion
d Parenchymal injury with haemorrhage without major duct disruption
e Post-traumatic pancreatitis

66 A patient presented with severe epigastric pain and acute severe pancreatitis was diagnosed. After resuscitation, what is the most useful first-line investigation in the first 24 hours?
a Triple-phase CT
b Dual-phase CT
c Plain abdominal radiograph
d Ultrasound abdomen
e MRI pancreas

67 A patient with pancreatitis underwent a CT scan. In addition to the expected CT findings of acute pancreatitis there was extensive pancreatic calcification and bilateral renal calculi and renal calcification. What underlying diagnosis does this suggest?
a Alcoholic pancreatitis
b Hyperparathyroidism
c Kwashiorkor
d Pancreatic carcinoma
e Sarcoid

68 A 70-year-old man gave a history of recurrent episodes of abdominal pain and weight loss. Ultrasound of the upper abdomen showed a non-specific abnormality for the pancreas and a CT was performed that demonstrated focal enlargement of the pancreatic head. The pancreas contained numerous irregular ductal calcifications and there was duct dilatation. There was no cystic change. What are these features most likely to represent?
a Chronic pancreatitis
b Cystic fibrosis
c Mucinous pancreatic neoplasm
d Pancreatic carcinoma
e Pancreatic islet cell tumour

69 An obese 55-year-old female had a history of abdominal bloating, but no other symptom was investigated. Plain chest and abdominal radiographs were normal. An ultrasound showed a moderate amount of ascites, but the views were limited and a contrast-enhanced CT was arranged which showed gross abdominal ascites with a mean density of 45 HU. No other abnormality was detected. What is most likely to have caused the ascites?

a Budd-Chiari syndrome

b Hypoalbuminaemia

c Meigs syndrome

d Right heart failure

e Unseen ovarian tumour

70 A four-month-old child presented with hyperpigmented wheal and flare skin lesions. An abdominal ultrasound showed hepatosplenomegaly and some enlarged retroperitoneal lymph nodes. Examination of the bowel showed ileal wall thickening and further investigations showed distorted thickened nodular folds in the ileum. What is the most likely diagnosis?

a Carcinoid

b Down syndrome

c Mastocytosis

d Phaeochromocytoma

e Trisomy 18

Cardiothoracic and vascular radiology

PAPER 1: ANSWERS AND EXPLANATIONS

1 Answer D: Aberrant left pulmonary artery

An aberrant right subclavian and aortic aneurysm cause posterior indentation. A right-sided aortic arch causes a right lateral indentation and a double arch is responsible for a 'reverse S', or impressions on both sides of the oesophagus.

2 Answer C: Rib notching

Rib notching is not seen in pseudocoarctation. This entity, once thought benign, is due to kinking of the aorta. Although there is no obstruction to flow, the abnormal anatomy can lead to aneurysmal dilatation distal to the abnormality.

3 Answer E: Atherosclerotic aortic aneurysm

A haematoma from a dissection is less likely to have a calcified rim and be in contact with the aorta. Given the history, an aortic aneurysm is most likely.

4 Answer B: Echocardiogram

The easiest and safest way to determine the presence and extent of pericardial fluid is with an echocardiogram.

5 Answer D: Takayasu's arteritis

The description is that of an arteritis, with oedema in the aortic wall on the STIR sequences. In a young adult, Takayasu's is the commonest large-vessel vasculitis.

6 Answer C: Polyarteritis nodosa

The angiogram findings are classic although not pathognomonic of PAN. With no history of SLE or rheumatoid it makes these less likely. Up to two-thirds of patients with PAN have bowel features of the disease.

7 Answer E: Hypertrophic cardiomyopathy

The location and pattern of enhancement is typical of this diagnosis. In amyloidosis the hyperenhancement is global and in sarcoidosis and myocarditis it affects the epicardial or mid-myocardial regions.

8 Answer A: Carney's Syndrome

Carney's Syndrome or Complex refers to a familial neoplastic lentiginous syndrome consisting of the following: primary pigmented nodular adrenocortical disease, lentigines, ephelides, blue nevi of the skin and mucosa, various tumours (including myxomas of the skin, heart and breast) and Sertoli-cells tumours of the testes.

9 Answer B: It is ideally used in a population with a low pre-test probability of coronary artery disease

It has a high negative predictive value and is ideally used in the population with a low pre-test probability of CAD as it prevents unnecessary invasive procedures. The Agatston scoring system is used to quantify coronary calcification.

10 Answer A: Chronic alcohol abuse

This is the most logical explanation for these appearances.

11 Answer C: Atrial septal defect

ASD is the most common presenting left to right shunt in adulthood.

12 Answer B: Myocardial infarction

Purely subendocardial delayed hyperenhancement in a recognised vascular territory is classical of myocardial infarction. The anteroseptal wall is supplied by the left anterior descending artery.

13 Answer C: SVCO secondary to metastatic bronchogenic carcinoma

Malignant lesions account for 80–90% of SVCO, and of these bronchogenic carcinoma accounts 50% of cases.

14 Answer E: Cardiac myxoma

The differential diagnosis of a pedunculated intracardiac lesion includes atrial myxoma and papillary fibroelastoma. Papillary fibroelastomas are rare lesions that are typically asymptomatic.

15 Answer B: Isolated diastolic dysfunction

One of the hallmarks of restrictive cardiomyopathy is diastolic dysfunction, whereas systolic dysfunction is typical of dilated cardiomyopathy. The presence of mural thrombus and increased LV cavity size can be seen in both forms of cardiomyopathy.

16 Answer A: Dextrocardia

The appearances are those of dextrocardia. Situs invertus describes reversal of the thoracic and abdominal organs in a mirror-image fashion. Situs solitus refers to normal orientation. Severe pectus excavatum can lead to an abnormal position of the heart towards the right of the midline; however, the ribs would have an abnormal orientation (horizontal posterior ribs and steeply sloping anterior ribs – the so-called '7' appearance).

17 Answer E: Takayasu's disease

Takayasu's disease causes granulomatous inflammation of large arteries. Polyarteritis nodosa affects medium-sized vessels. The other options are causes of small vessel vasculitis.

18 Answer C: Mitral stenosis

The description is most compatible with rheumatic mitral stenosis. Rheumatic heart disease usually develops 5–15 years after the initial episode of rheumatic fever. Other signs to consider include splaying of the carina and rightward displacement of the oesophagus on an oesophagram.

19 Answer A: Coils

Pulmonary arteriovenous malformation can be embolised with coils/balloons. There is a risk of embolisation to the systemic circulation with the other options

20 Answer D: High

With an acute myocardial infarction there will be a high intensity focus in the region of the infarcted tissue on T2-weighted imaging with no change or mildly decreased signal intensity on T1 due to myocardial oedema post infarction.

21 Answer B: Dobutamine

In patients with asthma or bronchospastic conditions, dobutamine can be used as a pharmacological stress agent. Dobutamine primarily acts on beta-1 receptors with its peak effect occurring within 10 minutes.

22 Answer A: First part of the artery, at its origin

In the subclavian steal syndrome, there is stenosis of the first part of the subclavian artery proximal to origin of the vertebral artery. The scalenus anterior muscle divides the subclavian artery into three parts.

23 Answer A: Aberrant left pulmonary artery

An aberrant left pulmonary artery arises from the right pulmonary artery and passes above the right main bronchus and between the trachea and oesophagus to reach the left lung. The right main stem bronchus may be bowed anteriorly and the trachea deviated to the left. There is an anterior indentation of the oesophagogram. Atelectasis and/or obstructive emphysema may be seen in the right (and/or left) upper lobe. It is associated with stenosis of the trachea, patent ductus arteriosus and absence of the pars membranacea.

24 Answer A: Left anterior descending artery

The left anterior descending artery is a branch of the left coronary artery and travels along the anterior interventricular groove. It usually supplies the anterior two-thirds of the interventricular septum and the posterior descending artery the posterior third of the septum.

25 Answer A: Bicuspid aortic valve

In the infantile form of aortic coarctation, there is a long segment of narrowing in the aortic arch after the origin of the innominate artery. Unlike the adult form, up to 50% have associated abnormalities. The most frequently associated abnormality is the bicuspid valve.

26 Answer C: Wait 4–6/52 after start of chemotherapy

Performing PET imaging after a procedure will produce inaccurate results as traumatised tissues have an increased metabolism and will mask any adjacent uptake due to pathology. Imaging should ideally wait six weeks post surgery, one week post biopsy, six weeks post chemotherapy and six months post radiation to avoid false positive uptake. However, some tumours such as GIST can show reduced metabolic activity and hence reduced uptake as soon as 24 hours following commencement of chemotherapy where conventional imaging will appear no different for weeks.

27 Answer C: Low probability

The Prospective Investigation of Pulmonary Embolus Diagnosis (PIOPED) criteria give a range of findings that can be reported, from normal study to high probability. The reporter should be familiar with the segmental anatomy and these criteria and the report should be taken into account along with the clinical probability.

28 Answer B: T2N1Mx

The satellite nodule would upstage this to M1 if positive but is too small to exclude this on PET, therefore metastatic disease cannot be accurately assessed and this should be mentioned in the report. The supraclavicular uptake sounds typical of brown fat uptake and providing there is no correlating soft tissue mass should be reported as such.

29 Answer B: Ventricular septal defect

This child has a ventricular septal defect (VSD) causing a left to right shunt and has right and left-sided cardiac enlargement (enlarged left atrium). Seventy-five to eighty per cent of VSDs are 'membranous' (opening in the upper section of the ventricular septum near the valves) and 10–15% are 'muscular' (opening in the lower section of the ventricular septum). Congestive heart failure rarely occurs in patients with PDA if the left to right shunt is large.

30 Answer A: Patent ductus arteriosus

In patent ductus arteriosus (PDA) there is a persistent connection between the left pulmonary artery and descending aorta. This causes increased volume of blood to flow from the aorta through the PDA to the pulmonary artery and lungs and then to the left atrium, resulting in left atrial and ventricular enlargement, bounding peripheral pulses, and a continuous murmur. The right ventricle may be enlarged with pulmonary hypertension.

31 Answer A: Anterior mediastinum

The Reed-Sternberg cell, although not common, is characteristic of Hodgkin's disease (which affects T-cells). The nodular sclerosing subtype is the most common and carries a relatively good prognosis. There is a bimodal distribution with peaks in the 25–30 and 75–80 age groups. Anterior mediastinal and retrosternal nodes are more commonly involved. The presence of a pleural effusion is not of prognostic significance.

32 Answer E: Adenocarcinoma

This is simply a question of incidence. It is the most common type of lung carcinoma and is also the most common in non-smokers.

33 Answer C: Gastric carcinoma

Ovarian carcinoma and extra hepatic bile duct carcinomas also demonstrate a high rate of pulmonary emboli.

34 Answer B: Pleural effusion

Pleural effusion is often the earliest abnormality in asbestos-related pleural disease but focal pleural plaques are more common during the later part of the disease. Very fine fibres such as crocidolite are more likely to result in extensive pleural disease.

35 Answer A: Pleural disease

Rheumatoid lung occurs more frequently in males with rheumatoid arthritis (although rheumatoid arthritis is more common in females). Pleural involvement is the most common thoracic manifestation while rheumatoid nodules are the rarest.

36 Answer C: Acute sarcoidosis

Features of acute sarcoidosis (Löfgren syndrome) include fever, malaise, bilateral hilar lymphadenopathy, erythema nodosum, arthralgia and occasionally parotitis and uveitis.

The Kveim-Siltzbach test is rarely used and involves intracutaneous injection of a suspension of human sarcoid spleen. ACE levels are more commonly used, which are elevated in 70% of sarcoid patients and are an indicator of the granuloma burden on the body.

37 Answer E: 150

38 Answer C: Allergic bronchopulmonary aspergillosis

This is classically described in patients with long-standing asthma and is the commonest cause of a pulmonary eosinophilia in the UK. The pulmonary infiltrates are often migratory and other key features include a finger-in-glove appearance of mucus plugs within dilated second-order bronchi.

39 Answer E: Drainage via pulmonary veins

The other findings are all more typical of an extralobar sequestration.

40 Answer D: Non-specific pneumonitis

The division between primary and secondary tuberculosis infection is not always clear-cut, as approximately 10% of primary infections progress uninterrupted into a more chronic progressive disease. It is generally accepted that the predominant radiological features of primary infections are adenopathy and foci of tuberculous pneumonitis (randomly distributed and ranging from small ill-defined airspace opacification to segmental and lobar consolidation).

41 Answer A: Pleural effusion

In both the acute and late-phases of EAA a normal chest radiograph is seen in 30–95%. No radiological study is pathognomonic, but appearances that would support a diagnosis include patchy non-specific pneumonitis, small pulmonary nodules (which may be so small they give the appearance of ground-glass consolidation) and more chronic changes reflecting healing fibrosis such as bronchiectasis and scarring. Although the horizontal fissure may become thickened, in general pleural disease is not a feature.

42 Answer B: Lymphangiomyomatosis

LAM is seen exclusively in women, typically those of child-bearing age. The typical appearances are of thin-walled cysts with normal intervening lung. There may also be small pneumothoraces and chylous effusions.

43 Answer B: Renal cell carcinoma

All these tumours except pancreatic carcinoma often metastasise to the chest but renal cell carcinoma is both the most common and the most likely to present with lung metastases already present.

44 Answer B: Incidence

Non-Hodgkin's lymphoma is approximately eight times more common than Hodgkin's lymphoma. Hodgkin's lymphoma is a disease solely of T-cells as opposed to non-Hodgkin's lymphoma which can involve T or B cells. Adenopathy most commonly involves the anterior mediastinal nodes. Pleural effusion is non-discriminatory.

45 Answer C: Kaposi's sarcoma

Lymphoma, histoplasmosis, *Pneumocystis* and CMV are all usually seen when the CD4 count is below 200.

46 Answer A: Nodular interlobular septal thickening

In lymphangitis carcinomatosis the interlobular septal thickening is caused by tumour infiltration and is more often irregular or nodular in appearance. The remaining features would not be unusual in either condition.

47 Answer E: Silicosis

All the other conditions would produce nodules of soft tissue density. In pure silicosis the nodules are very well defined and very dense. There is also relative sparing of the bases and apices with septal lines on HRCT.

48 Answer B: Predominantly dependent abnormality

Almost all patients with ARDS will have bilateral dependent abnormalities. Ground-glass attenuation is seen but in less than 10%. Pneumothorax and pneumatoceles are uncommon.

49 Answer C: Compression of the phrenic nerve by a tumour

This is largely a question of probability, as the clinical history is non-specific. A tumour causing compression is the commonest cause in adults.

50 Answer D: Cryptogenic organising pneumonia

These imaging findings are classical of COP. Effusions and adenopathy are also present in up to one-third of patients. Bronchoalveolar cell carcinoma is an important differential, but is most commonly solitary and centrilobular nodules are not a feature, and there is a strong smoking association.

51 Answer A: Wegener's granulomatosis

The clinical differential diagnosis is between Wegener's granulomatosis and Goodpasture's syndrome and the imaging findings are classical for Wegener's granulomatosis. Findings in Goodpasture's syndrome include consolidation with relative apical sparing in the acute stage, followed by an interstitial pattern of opacification in the later stages of the disease.

52 Answer D: Dilution of opacified blood with unopacified blood

This is a common problem with the CTPA, especially with younger patients. As they take in a deep breath just prior to the scan their intrathoracic pressure is reduced and unopacified blood is drawn up from the IVC. This effectively dilutes the opacified blood entering from the SVC. One way to avoid this pitfall is to ask the patient to only take a modest breath prior to scanning.

53 Answer A: Middle lobe collapse

The findings are those of middle lobe collapse. Signs on the frontal radiograph can be subtle, and it is more easily seen on the lateral radiograph. In this case the loss of clarity of the right atrial border indicates the pathology is located in the middle lobe. There is loss of volume (the normal horizontal fissure runs from the hilum to the sixth rib in the mid axillary line), therefore collapse of the middle lobe, rather than consolidation, is the likely cause for these appearances.

54 Answer C: Isolated homogeneous soft tissue mass within the anterior mediastinum outlined by fat

The neurological findings are classic of the myasthenia gravis – an autoimmune disorder characterised by antibodies against postjunctional acetylcholine receptors. The condition is often associated with thymoma.

55 Answer D: Honeycombing

Reduced lung volumes, septal thickening and traction bronchiectasis are features of both conditions. Honeycombing is more prevalent in UIP, but can be seen in NSIP. A consistent finding in NSIP is relatively symmetrical, basal ground glass-opacification due to cellular infiltrate. The presence of ground-glass opacification on HRCT in UIP usually represents fine interstitial fibrosis, beyond the resolving power of HRCT rather than a potentially reversible cellular infiltrate. NSIP has been linked to connective tissue diseases such as scleroderma.

56 Answer D: Lymphoid interstitial infiltrate

Lymphoid interstitial pneumonitis (LIP) is characterised by a widespread interstitial lymphoid infiltrate, resembling lymphoma but with a clinical course more in keeping with a chronic interstitial pneumonia. LIP is more common in women than in men. Frequently, patients with LIP have evidence of an abnormal immune response such as Sjögren's disease or AIDS.

57 Answer C: Bilateral focal pleural thickening predominantly affecting the diaphragms and lower thorax, sparing the apices, costophrenic angles and mediastinal pleura. Only a few of the plaques are calcified.

The typical appearances of benign asbestos-related pleural plaques are bilateral focal pleural thickening of the chest wall between the seventh and tenth ribs and diaphragms with sparing of the costophrenic angles, apices and mediastinal pleura. Plaques show a predilection for the posterior-lateral portion of the chest wall and may or may not be calcified. Appearances raising the possibility of malignant mesothelioma include concentric pleural thickening involving the mediastinal pleura, pleural effusion and effacement of the subpleural fat plane.

58 Answer E: Alveolar proteinosis

Alveolar proteinosis (AP) is a rare condition predominantly affecting men. Symptoms are non-specific. It is caused by altered surfactant homeostasis leading to accumulation of lipoproteinacious material within the alveoli. AP affects the airspaces only, and not the interstitium, and is a rare cause for a 'crazy paving' pattern on HRCT.

59 Answer C: Severe upper zone bullous emphysema with relatively spared lower zones.

Lung volume reduction surgery (LVRS) is a palliative procedure for patients with advanced disease. It has a number of clinical exclusion criteria because of relatively high operative risk. There are still some controversies around this form of surgery, but it is likely to continue to have a place in the treatment of emphysema. It comprises wedge resection of the areas of greatest disease, mainly the upper lobes, thus improving the performance of the remaining lung. Best candidates for surgery have upper lobe predominant emphysema, a good amount of normal or mildly emphysematous lung and significant regional heterogeneity on perfusion scintigraphy.

60 Answer E: Septated effusion with underlying consolidation on ultrasound. Biochemical/cytological analysis: ph 7.1, neutrophils ++

Ultrasound is useful for delineating small effusions that may not be easily appreciated on plain radiography. Typical features of an infected effusion (empyema) on ultrasound are the presence of reflective debris and septations, although the absence of these findings does not exclude empyema. Pathological analysis of the fluid is needed to confirm or refute the presence of an empyema. Typically the ph is <7.3, glucose is low, LDH is raised and neutrophils are present.

61 Answer B: Fat embolism

Fat embolism is caused by obstruction of pulmonary vessels by fat globules following major skeletal trauma. Onset is typically 24–48 hours following trauma. The CXR is often normal in the acute phase, progressing to consolidation and atelectasis thereafter.

62 Answer E: Acute transplant rejection

The clinical picture is that of acute rejection within the lung transplant. This condition usually responds to high-dose intravenous steroids. Bronchiolitis obliterans syndrome (i.e. chronic rejection) is an obliterative bronchiolitis that develops in transplanted lung after three months. Findings include air trapping, mosaic perfusion and bronchiectasis.

63 Answer A: Call for the resuscitation team

Reactions to iodinated contrast include: nausea/vomiting, bronchospasm, laryngeal oedema, hypotension, generalised anaphylactoid reaction, contrast medium extravasation and delayed skin reactions. The symptoms described are of a generalised anaphylactoid reaction.

Royal College of Radiologists. *Standards for Iodinated Intravascular Contrast Agent Administration to Adult Patients*. London: RCR; 2005.

64 Answer C: 10 mL

Lidocaine hydrochloride (xylocaine, lignocaine) is routinely used for local anaesthesia. 1% means 1 g in 100 mL, that is 10 mg/mL. In a typical adult a maximum dose of 3 mg/kg is appropriate. (In solutions containing adrenaline, the maximum dose is higher: 7 mg/kg.)

65 Answer A: Normal transplant

Resistive index (RI) (also known as the resistivity or Pourcelot index) is a useful vascular parameter in assessing renal and other transplants. It is based on the ratio between peak systolic velocity and end diastolic flow. RI of less than 0.8 is taken as normal. Almost any parenchymal renal process will make the kidney 'tighter' and therefore increase RI.

66 Answer D: 18 Fr

The French Catheter Scale is used to grade the circumference of catheters. The French size is equivalent to three times the diameter in millimetres. Thus a 6-mm lumen will accept an 18 Fr catheter.

67 Answer C: Superficial femoral artery

Atherosclerotic disease typically has a symmetrical pattern and develops at points of turbulent flow (e.g. bifurcations). In the lower limb the commonly affected sites are: SFA > Iliac artery > Tibial artery > Popliteal artery > CFA.

68 Answer D: Polyarteritis nodosa

Renal artery aneurysms can be broadly divided into extrarenal and intrarenal. Extrarenal causes include atherosclerosis and fibromuscular dysplasia. Intrarenal aneurysms are usually due to polyarteritis nodosa (PAN). Pan is a rare necrotising vasculitis that affects small and medium-sized arteries of multiple organs. The kidney and liver are most commonly affected. Patients may also develop characteristic subcutaneous nodules.

69 Answer E: Popliteal entrapment

In popliteal entrapment the popliteal artery is displaced medially around the medial head of gastrocnemius. It is common in young athletes, and should be considered in leg ischaemia without trauma in this age group.

70 Answer B: Type II endoleak

Endoleaks are common immediately post EVAR and most resolve spontaneously. They are classified as follows:
I Leak from proximal or distal graft attachment site
II Retrograde filling of sac from persistent collateral vessel
III Leak from midgraft/component junction
IV Leak through porous graft material
V Endotension

Cardiothoracic and vascular radiology

PAPER 2: ANSWERS AND EXPLANATIONS

1   Answer C: Indistinct aortic arch contour

2   Answer C: A persistent left superior vena cava

A persistent left superior vena cava (SVC) courses along the left mediastinal border and enters the coronary sinus, which is usually dilated. There is more often than not a right SVC as well.

3   Answer B: Ebstein's anomaly

The description is that of Ebstein's anomaly. Tricuspid atresia would not have a functioning right ventricle.

4   Answer B: Mitral valve stenosis

The description is that of left atrial enlargement and with the calcification of the left atrium, this is most in keeping with mitral stenosis.

5   Answer D: Intravenously in Eisenmenger's syndrome

Carbon dioxide is a useful negative vascular contrast agent in situations where iodinated contrast is contraindicated. The main risk is cerebral toxicity and it should therefore be avoided intra-arterially above the diaphragm and intravenously in patients with a right-to-left shunt.

6   Answer D: Atherosclerosis

Popliteal artery entrapment is a rare cause of occlusive disease and is classically seen in young men. Atherosclerosis is a common condition and although it is unusual to affect the popliteal region with comparative sparing elsewhere, it would still be the most likely cause in an older smoker.

7   Answer D: Right coronary artery

The right coronary artery supplies the posterior descending artery responsible for supplying the inferior wall in 85% of people. The circumflex is responsible in 10%. Co-dominance is responsible for the remaining 5%.

8 Answer C: Arrhythmogenic right ventricular dysplasia (ARVD)

This is an uncommon disease which is often familial. It is characterised by the replacement of the myocardium by fatty and fibrous tissue. The commonest symptoms are syncopal episodes or sudden death. MRI has the advantage over echocardiography that it demonstrates the presence of fat as well as fibrous tissue on delayed enhancement imaging.

9 Answer C: An aneurysm that protruded only in systole

Although most true aneurysms protrude in diastole and systole, a functional aneurysm protrudes only in systole. All false aneurysms protrude in diastole and systole.

10 Answer B: Left internal mammary artery

The distal left anterior descending (LAD) artery lies anteriorly in the chest. The left internal mammary artery (LIMA) lies along the anterior chest wall and passes close to the LAD in the interventricular groove, which makes it an ideal graft. Additionally, arteries make more sustainable graft material.

11 Answer C: Mosaic attenuation

Mosaic attenuation is a common feature of chronic thromboembolism; it can be seen in left to right shunts but this is much less common and tends to be more diffuse.

12 Answer E: Tako-tsubo cardiomyopathy

This description is classic of Tako-tsubo cardiomyopathy, which is also known as transient catecholaminergic myocardial stunning. It often occurs following a stressful event and most patients recover completely.

13 Answer E: Stanford type B

The Stanford classification of aortic dissection determines management of aortic dissection. Type B dissections involve only the descending aorta and are usually treated non-surgically. Type A dissections always involve the ascending aorta. They may also involve a variable portion of the arch and descending aorta. Type A dissections are managed surgically.

14 Answer C: Echocardiography

In the presence of a deep-vein thrombosis (DVT) an embolic stroke raised through a right to left shunt should be investigated. Under certain circumstances, for example during temporary raised intrathoracic pressure when lifting a heavy shopping bag, in the presence of an atrial septal defect (ASD) or ventricular septal defect (VSD), emboli may cross from the venous to arterial circulation. Therefore, in this case the search for a cardiac septal defect (most likely to be an ASD) with echocardiography is indicated.

15 Answer B: Ventricular septal defect (VSD)

The following features can differentiate between the position of acyanotic shunts:

Lesion	Chamber enlargement	Dilated aorta
ASD	Right atrium	No
	Right ventricle	
VSD	Left atrium	No
	Left ventricle	
	Right ventricle	
PDA	Left atrium	Yes
	Left Ventricle	

16 Answer E: Loss of phasic flow on Valsalva

Direct evidence of thrombus: Inability to compress the vein with transducer pressure, intraluminal echogenic thrombus (acute clot may be poorly echogenic), increased luminal diameter in acute thrombus, reduced diameter in chronic thrombus, vein wall thickening and absent flow in occlusive thrombus.

Indirect evidence of thrombus: Loss of phasic flow with respiration/Valsalva suggesting proximal venous obstruction, loss of venous distension on Valsalva, minimal increase in flow on squeezing the calf, increased flow in superficial veins and deep collaterals.

17 Answer A: Tricuspid valve endocarditis and septic pulmonary emboli

Intravenous drug abusers are prone to right-sided valvular endocarditis from organisms introduced to the venous system while injecting. These vegetations, seen most commonly on the tricuspid valve, often throw off emboli to the lungs.

18 Answer A: Congenital bicuspid aortic valve

The murmur description is consistent with aortic stenosis. In an otherwise young and healthy individual, a congenital bicuspid aortic valve is most likely. These individuals can become clinically symptomatic under the age of 30. Aortic valve calcification is a not uncommon finding on the chest radiograph. Atherosclerotic disease of the aortic valve presents later in life. Rheumatic aortic valve disease is rare in the absence of mitral valve disease.

19 Answer E: 25 mmHg

The above vignette describes pulmonary hypertension. The normal pulmonary arterial pressure is about 15 mmHg at rest and it is considered elevated if it measures above 25 mmHg.

20   Answer E: 10–15 minutes

The ECG findings are consistent with inferior myocardial infarction within the right coronary artery territory. A perfusion defect will occur within 60–90 seconds after contrast administration. There will be delayed enhancement of the infarcted tissue, which is most visible at 10–15 minutes. The size of the enhanced area correlates well with the size of the infarction.

21   Answer C: Ostium secundum atrial septal defect

Atrial septal defects are one of the most common congenital cardiac defects. Ostium secundum defects account for the majority (70%) of ASDs, ostium primum defects for 20–25%. ASDs often present in the third or fourth decade and the most frequent reported symptoms are breathlessness and fatigue on exertion. Patients may develop cardiac arrhythmias and the risk of thromboembolism is increased due to the presence of arrhythmias and the possibility of paradoxical embolus.

22   Answer D: Left vertebral artery

In subclavian steal syndrome there is flow reversal in the ipsilateral vertebral artery at the expense of the cerebral circulation. This can be confirmed with colour Doppler imaging or MR. The condition is usually secondary to atherosclerosis and males are more commonly affected. The condition is three times as common on the left. Angioplasty yields good long-term results but some individuals require bypass surgery.

23   Answer C: Right cardiophrenic angle

Pericardial cysts may develop as a sequelae of pericarditis. The majority of these lesions are located in the cardiophrenic angle and are three times more common on the right. Occasionally, they may occur in the mediastinum. They can change in shape and size with respiration and body position.

24   Answer A: Type I

In a type I endoleak, there is blood flow into the aneurysm sac due to incomplete seal or ineffective seal at the end of the graft. This type of endoleak usually occurs in the early course of treatment, but may also occur later.

25   Answer E: The dominant annihilation photon interaction in tissue is Compton scatter

The range of resolution of positron emission tomography is 5–10 mm, much less than that of CT which can resolve points of less than 1 mm, which limits its use in detecting sub-5 mm lesions. F-18 is a positron emitter (hence positron emission tomography) and has a half-life of 109 minutes. During FDG positron decay the nuclide decays into a proton and neutron with the emission of a positron with a range of approximately 1 mm. This interacts with an electron to produce two annihilation photons (511 keV) travelling in opposite directions. These photons form the images of tracer concentration.

26   Answer E: Increase in diastolic blood pressure above 120 mmHg

Most patients experience mildly unpleasant symptoms during chemical stressing with adenosine or dobutamine. These should all be documented and can be correlated with any induced ECG changes. Obviously, the procedure should be stopped at the patient's request but forewarning about possible side-effects is helpful. ST segment depression of >3 mm is an indication to stop. Systolic decrease is also worrying but should be taken into account with any concurrent symptoms.

27   Answer A: Tc Myoview rest and chemical stress

Cardiac gated CT is useful to assess anatomy and can be used for coronary calcification scoring. It will not demonstrate ischaemia. MR studies with stress can demonstrate myocardial ischaemia and contractility but are usually used for those with complex disease or anatomy. The atypical symptoms make her more appropriate for a nuclear medicine study. She would probably struggle with an exercise tolerance test and a resting only study would not show reversible ischaemia.

28   Answer C: Reduced-dose ventilation/perfusion scan

Ventilation/perfusion scans (V/Q) are considered the best form of imaging in pregnancy, especially in a fit patient with no chest disease. A reduced-dose study enables both perfusion and ventilation images to be performed at less than the conventional dose. A MUGA study looks at ejection fraction; cardiac echo may show evidence of right heart strain and large central PE but will not exclude segmental disease.

29   Answer D: 67

The median is the middle of the dataset. If there is an even number of data points then the median is the average of the middle two. The mode is the most frequently occurring number and the arithmetic mean is the sum of all the values divided by the number of data points included.

30   Answer B: Lymphangiomyomatosis

Lymphangiomyomatosis is a rare condition seen exclusively in women of childbearing age. It is characterised by gradual progressive interstitial disease, recurrent pneumothoraces and chylous pleural effusions. The key feature is the presence of numerous thin-walled cysts of varying sizes diffusely scattered throughout the lungs with normal intervening lung parenchyma. In histiocytosis cysts are located in the upper two-thirds of the lungs, walls are of varying thickness and septal thickening is usually present. In neurofibromatosis, the cystic spaces are predominantly located in the lung apices.

31   Answer C: Stage III

Ann Arbor classification is most commonly used. In stage I disease, there is involvement of one or two contiguous regions on the same side of the diaphragm. In stage II disease, more than two contiguous regions are involved on the same side of the diaphragm. When there is disease on both sides of the diaphragm, it is classed as stage III. Stage IV disease indicates organ involvement. The thymus and spleen are considered a 'lymph node' in staging.

32 Answer C: Similar to skeletal muscle

Thymomas are the most common primary tumour of the anterior mediastinum and half are detected incidentally. The remainder may demonstrate symptoms secondary to mediastinal compression. Malignant thymomas tend to show changes in the mediastinal fat and fascial planes.

33 Answer D: Hydatid

34 Answer B: Bronchoalveolar cell carcinoma

Lung carcinoma is more frequent in individuals with asbestos exposure (20–25% lifetime risk) and bronchoalveolar carcinoma is the most common subtype. Smoking further increases the risk. The risk of malignant mesothelioma is 10% over the lifetime of an asbestos worker, with a 20- to 40-year latency period.

35 Answer D: Bases

Interstitial fibrosis is most common in the lower lobes. In early pulmonary disease, reticulonodular densities are seen and become progressively coarser in the later stages.

36 Answer C: Carcinoid

Pulmonary carcinoid is a slow-growing low-grade malignant vascular tumour. It is often centrally located (70–90%). Up to one-third of these calcify but cavitation is rare. Pulmonary carcinoid rarely results in the carcinoid syndrome. It commonly shows no tracer uptake on PET imaging. It is occasionally associated with MEN type I.

37 Answer A: Breast

38 Answer B: Bronchiolitis obliterans

This is defined as inflammation of the bronchioles leading to obstruction of the lumen and is seen in patients with cystic fibrosis, connective tissue disorders, post-infection, in transplanted lungs, following inhaled toxins, drug therapy (methotrexate, bleomycin, cyclophosphamide, penicillamine), but can be idiopathic.

39 Answer C: Cystic fibrosis

Hyperinflation and peribronchial thickening are non-specific signs and could be seen in asthma or aspergillosis, but the further imaging findings make asthma unlikely and the organisms grown make aspergillosis and TB less likely. Patients with cystic fibrosis are more susceptible to pseudomonas infections.

40 Answer C: Diffuse bronchiectasis and centrilobular nodulation

In the majority of cases the two organisms produce virtually indistinguishable radiological features. The history of COPD in an elderly woman should raise the possibility of MAI, and in this subset of patients diffuse bronchiectasis and centrilobular nodules are suggestive of the diagnosis. In favour of tuberculosis is the greater incidence of interlobular septal thickening. Often the failure of response to antituberculous therapy leads to the consideration of MAI.

41 Answer C: Advise no further investigations necessary. The most likely diagnosis is a pulmonary hamartoma

The presence of fat attenuation in a lung mass is diagnostic of a pulmonary hamartoma. Chondroid ('popcorn') calcification is another diagnostic feature.

42 Answer B: Chronic eosinophilic pneumonia

Alveolar infiltrates in a peripheral distribution can also be seen in resolving pulmonary oedema, desquamative interstitial pneumonia and sarcoidosis.

43 Answer B: Malignant mesothelioma

It is associated with pleural plaques in only about 50% of cases. Pleural effusions are common and can often be large enough to obscure the underlying tumour. A useful differentiator from other causes of pleural effusion is the lack of shift of midline structures as the mediastinum is fixed by the disease process.

44 Answer D. Linear densities radiating from the edge of the lesion into the surrounding lung

Although not specific for malignancy, a spiculated margin is highly suspicious. This represents reoriented connective tissue drawn into the tumour by the cicatrising nature of many malignant tumours. There are benign processes that can cause this appearance such as lipoid pneumonias and tuberculomas, but the remaining features are more likely to suggest a benign aetiology.

45 Answer D: T3, N2, M0

The current TNM staging system is set to change in January 2010, but this answer remains correct according to the proposed revisions for the 7th edition. The new staging provides a more comprehensive breakdown of tumour size and a change in the classification of separate tumour nodules.

46 Answer A: Pleural effusion

All of these are found in rheumatoid lung disease but the commonest is a unilateral pleural effusion with no other pulmonary changes. On aspiration the fluid is an exudate with a low white cell count (high in lymphocytes) and a low glucose.

47 Answer A: Bronchiectasis

As a late complication of viral bronchiolitis in childhood, bronchiectasis is the most correct answer. On V/Q scan a matched defect is seen in the affected areas, and the ipsilateral vessels and hilar are small.

48 Answer D: Asthma

Even though the chest radiograph is normal and he was previously fit and well, asthma is by far the commonest and therefore most likely answer.

49 Answer D: Radiation pneumonitis

The location and well-defined margin are typical of post-radiation damage to the lung. Breast cancer is routinely treated with radiotherapy.

50 Answer E: Sarcoidosis

This constellation of symptoms and bi-hilar adenopathy, in the absence of parenchymal changes, is typical of acute sarcoid – Löfgren syndrome.

51 Answer D: Usual interstitial pneumonia (UIP)

These are the classical HRCT findings in established pulmonary fibrosis. The lower-zone subpleural distribution is typical of UIP. The other diagnoses here have an upper-zone predilection.

52 Answer D: Reactivation tuberculosis

The description of interconnected subpleural nodules is that of 'tree-in-bud'. This represents bronchiolar luminal impaction with mucus, pus or fluid. The causes are myriad (in fact all the options are potential causes). Infection is the commonest cause, and tuberculosis (via endobronchial spread) is the commonest infection accounting for this appearance.

53 Answer E: Pulmonary arteriovenous malformation

Orthodeoxia describes worsening hypoxia in the erect position due to gravitational shift of blood within the arteriovenous malformation (AVM). Seventy per cent of AVMs are located in the lower lobes, and small foci of calcification may be seen within them, representing phleboliths. The cordlike bands seen connecting the AVM to the hilum represent the feeding artery and draining vein.

54 Answer A: Fibrosing mediastinitis

The findings are classical of fibrosing mediastinitis. The most common presentation is that of a focal mass lesion containing calcification causing compression of the pulmonary vasculature leading to right heart strain, peribronchial cuffing, septal thickening and wedge-shaped areas of pulmonary infarction. There is an association with retroperitoneal fibrosis and orbital pseudotumour.

55 Answer B: Respiratory bronchiolitis-associated interstitial lung disease (RBILD)

RBILD is seen almost exclusively in heavy smokers. Centrilobular nodules are a key finding, and are not commonly seen in other interstitial pneumonitides, except LIP, where air trapping is not such a prominent feature. The histology and aetiology of RBILD and desquamative interstitial pneumonia (DIP) are very similar and they may represent the ends of a spectrum of a single disease.

56 Answer E: Nodular thickening of the fissures

Pleural effusions are rare in both conditions and the remaining options are features of both sarcoid and EAA. The nodules in sarcoid, seen along broncho-arterial bundles and veins and within septal lymphatics, are caused by epitheliod cell granulomas.

57 Answer A: Silicosis

Pneumoconiosis is caused by the inhalation and deposition of fine particles of inorganic dust in the lungs. The inhaled dust may be classified as non-fibrogenic or fibrogenic, depending on how the body reacts to the inhaled particles. Coal, tin (stannosis) and iron oxide (siderosis) are non-fibrogenic, whereas silica and beryllium are fibrogenic. The clinical and radiological picture here is one of fibrosis caused by long-term silica dust inhalation. Hilar lymph node eggshell calcification is very typical of silicosis.

58 Answer A: Post-intubation stricture

The findings are those of a short tracheal stricture. The most common cause for a discrete stricture is a traumatic insult, in this case likely to be due to the balloon cuff from an endotracheal tube. Other causes of tracheal strictures include previous radiotherapy or surgery and burns.

59 Answer C: Kaposi's sarcoma

Kaposi's sarcoma tends to affect patients whose CD4 count has fallen below 200. *Pneumocystis carinii* pneumonia is the commonest cause of opportunistic pulmonary infection in HIV, but the presence of characteristic skin lesions confirms the diagnosis in this instance. Imaging features of *Pneumocystis carinii* pneumonia include bilateral ground-glass infiltrates, interstitial infiltrates and pneumatoceles. Adenopathy and effusions are rarely seen.

60 Answer C: Aspiration pneumonia

The blood tests point to chronic alcohol excess. Acute alcohol intoxication is a common cause of aspiration. The clue as to the diagnosis lies in the predominantly dependent distribution of changes and relative sparing of the left lung.

61 Answer E: Churg-Strauss disease

Churg-Strauss disease is a multi-system disease and is a variant of polyarteritis nodosa. It is characterised by rhinitis, asthma, peripheral blood eosinophilia and a systemic small-vessel granulomatous vasculitis. Clinical manifestations are caused by a necrotising vasculitis, eosinophilic tissue invasion and extravascular granulomatous eosinophilic abscesses. The imaging findings within the lungs are those of pulmonary haemorrhage and eosinophilic pneumonia.

62 Answer A: Reperfusion syndrome

The acute onset (within 48 hours) and lack of fluid overload indicate a diagnosis of reperfusion oedema over acute rejection and cardiogenic pulmonary oedema respectively. Reperfusion syndrome is due to increased permeability due to lymphatic disruption, ischemia, trauma and pulmonary denervation. It is the most common immediate post-operative complication following lung transplantation.

63 Answer D: Obesity

There are a number of factors that increase the risk of femoral pseudoaneurysm formation:

Procedural factors: interventional rather than diagnostic procedures, catheterisation of artery and vein and catheterisation of SFA or profunda. Poor technique: low femoral puncture and inadequate compression post procedure.

Patient factors include: obesity, anticoagulation, haemodialysis and calcified arteries.

64 Answer D: Percutaneous thrombin injection

It is likely the patient has a false femoral aneurysm following a percutaneous intervention.

Ahmad F, Turner SA, Torrie P, *et al*. Iatrogenic femoral artery pseudoaneurysms: a review of current methods of diagnosis and treatment. *Clin Radiol*. 2008; **63**(12): 1310–16.

65 Answer A: 200 mg IV bolus over 15 seconds followed by 100 mg at one-minute intervals up to a maximum of 1000 mg

Midazolam is a short-acting benzodiazepine and is widely used in interventional procedures. It should be used with particular caution in the elderly, where it is more likely to cause respiratory depression and agitation. Flumazenil (Anexate®) reverses the action of midazolam and other benzodiazepines. An infusion of 100–400 mg/hr can be used for longer-acting benzodiazepines but, for rapid reversal, an initial 200-mg bolus is most appropriate.

66 Answer D: Reduce episodes of pulmonary oedema

The role of angioplasty and stenting in renal artery stenosis is controversial. The preliminary results of the ASTRAL (Angioplasty and STent for Renal Artery Lesions) trial show that stenting offers no benefit above medical treatment in terms of hypertension, renal function or mortality. It is likely that in hypertensive patients, with preserved left ventricular function, stenting reduces episodes of 'flash' non-cardiogenic pulmonary oedema.

67 Answer C: Gelfoam

Temporary embolic agents include: autologous blood clot and gelfoam. Permanent agents include: ethyl alcohol, steel coils, polyvinyl alcohol and glue. New embolic agents are frequently being introduced and this is, by no means, an exhaustive list.

68 Answer E: Severe right-sided heart failure

The only absolute contraindications to TIPS are severe right-sided heart failure with elevated central venous pressure and polycystic liver disease. Relative contraindications include active infection, severe encephalopathy, portal vein thrombosis, hypervascular liver tumours and hepatic failure.

69 Answer E: String-of-beads appearance

Fibromuscular dysplasia most commonly manifests as a 'string-of-beads' appearance in the renal artery and responds well to PTA. Atherosclerotic renal artery disease is less amenable to PTA although mid renal artery stenoses respond better than ostial stenoses.

70 Answer E: The patient received streptokinase 10 years ago

Contraindications to thrombolysis include: recent trauma, surgery or CPR (within two weeks), brain tumour or CVA within two months, bleeding tendency, irreversible limb ischaemia and pregnancy.

Cardiothoracic and vascular radiology

PAPER 3: ANSWERS AND EXPLANATIONS

1 Answer E: A narrowed superior mediastinum

The foetal circulation enables normal haemodynamics and affected infants often have a normal birth weight. Cardiomegaly then develops one to two weeks after birth. The aortic arch is small and the heart has a typically 'egg-on-its side' appearance caused by the narrow superior mediastinum and abnormal relationship of the vessels. The pulmonary trunk is absent in 99% of cases and the pulmonary arteries are located in the midline.

2 Answer B: Tetralogy of Fallot

Cardiomegaly would be expected with Ebstein's anomaly. The remaining options would have increased pulmonary venous flow.

3 Answer D: A pericardial cyst

A pericardial cyst typically occurs in the cardiophrenic angle and is characteristically low signal on T1-weighted MRI.

4 Answer A: A pericardial thickness on CT of 4 mm

Although pericardial thickening does not confirm a diagnosis of constrictive pericarditis, when the differential is between that and a restrictive cardiomyopathy it favours the former. B, C and D are non-discriminatory. E is occasionally found in restrictive cardiomyopathy.

5 Answer D: 33 mm

Usually a stent is oversized by approximately 10% to ensure a seal.

6 Answer C: No myocardial delayed enhancement

Hibernation describes chronic contractile impairment secondary to chronic hypoperfusion, where the myocardium is still viable. Delayed hyperenhancement represents infarcted tissue, which is no longer viable.

7   Answer C: Rhabdomyoma

The commonest cardiac tumour in an infant is a rhabdomyoma. It is a hamartoma and therefore a benign tumour that in 50–80% of patients is associated with tuberous sclerosis. They are often multiple and usually involve the ventricular free walls or interventricular septum. They are only managed surgically if they cause obstruction of the outflow tract as they tend to regress over time.

8   Answer B: Atrial septal defect

The enlarged heart and pulmonary plethora suggest a left to right shunt. At this age the only likely cause is an ASD.

9   Answer A: Pulmonary stenosis

A VSD, transposition of the great vessels and truncus arteriosus would usually produce pulmonary plethora and Tetralogy of Fallot would have a normal-sized heart.

10   Answer A: A contour deformity on the inner aortic wall at the level of the isthmus

Aortic transection occurs most commonly (90%) at the isthmus, typically presenting as a contour deformity.

11   Answer D: Cardiac vein

This appearance describes a cardiac resynchronisation pacemaker, used for cardiac failure in the presence of bundle branch block. The lead enters the coronary sinus from the right atrium then is placed within an appropriate cardiac vein adjacent to left ventricular myocardium. If cardiac venous anatomy is not suitable then surgically placed epicardial leads can be used.

12   Answer A: Right coronary artery arising from the left coronary sinus and passing anterior to the aorta

This arterial course is between aorta and pulmonary artery, which can compress the vessel causing ischaemia and if symptomatic may require bypass surgery. The commonest anomalous coronary artery course is an aberrant circumflex arising from the right coronary and passing posteriorly into the left AV groove (option c).

13   Answer A: Saccular aneurysm of the ascending aorta with thin, dystrophic wall calcification

This is the typical description of a syphilitic aneurysm. Options B, C, D and E are typical of a mycotic aneurysm, an atherosclerotic aneurysm, an inflammatory aneurysm and an actively leaking aneurysm respectively.

14   Answer E: Left ventricular outflow narrowing

Both conditions can be inherited. Options a) and b) are typical of ARVD. Aortic dilatation is not a feature of either disease. Other imaging findings in HCM include mitral regurgitation, systolic anterior motion of the anterior leaflet to the mitral valve (SAM), hyperkinetic left ventricular free wall, hypokinetic interventricular septum and early closure of the aortic valve.

15 Answer D: Focal myocardial fibrosis

The clinical scenario is one of acute myocardial infarction. The echocardiographic findings are those of a regional wall motion abnormality, which may be due to established infarction and scar formation, ischemia without infarction or aneurysm. The MRI findings are those of delayed hyperenhancement indicating an area of fibrosis/scarring due to the previous infarct. Viable myocardium will transiently enhance, but non-viable infarcted myocardium accumulates contrast and demonstrates high signal at 10–20 minutes.

16 Answer C: Inferior border third and fourth ribs

In localised (adult type) coarctation there is usually a short segment of narrowing near the ligamentum arteriosum. These patients may present with headaches due to hypertension and lower limb claudication secondary to poor perfusion. Rib notching develops due to enlarged and tortuous intercostal arteries. It involves the inferior aspect of the central and lateral thirds of the posterior ribs and is most pronounced in ribs three and four. The first two ribs are usually spared because their intercostal arteries originate from the subclavian arteries. Rib notching is commonly bilateral but may be unilateral in the presence of an aberrant subclavian artery.

17 Answer B: Superior vena cava

Partial anomalous pulmonary venous return (PAPVR) is a congenital abnormality, which can be radiologically mistaken for an anomalous SVC. One or more pulmonary veins drain directly into the right atrium or to a systemic vein. In decreasing order of frequency, the sites of communications are to the SVC, right atrium and IVC. This results in an extracardiac left to right shunt. The clinical signs and symptoms are related to the degree of left-to-right shunting. Although an isolated PAPVR from a single lobe is usually asymptomatic, individuals with cardiopulmonary disease may develop symptoms.

Burney K, Young H, Barnard S, *et al*. CT appearances of congenital and abnormalities of the SVC. *Clin Radiol*. 2007; **62**: 837–42.

18 Answer D: Hereditary haemorrhagic telangiectasia

Hereditary haemorrhagic telangiectasia is also known as Osler-Weber-Rendu syndrome and often presents with recurrent bleeding episodes (epistaxis, GI bleeding). It is the only condition of the options listed that is associated with pulmonary arteriovenous malformation (PAVM) and 50–60% of patients with PAVM have hereditary haemorrhagic telangiectasia. Ten to fifteen per cent of patients with hereditary haemorrhagic telangiectasia have PAVMs. With PAVMs, there is an extra-cardiac right-to-left shunt, which can result in paradoxical embolism. Brain abscesses can occur due to the loss of the normal pulmonary filter function. Screening first-degree relatives of patients with PAVMs is usually recommended as it is autosomally dominantly inherited.

19 Answer D: Immediate surgery.

The patient has a Stanford type A aortic dissection, which is associated with a high mortality and medical management alone is insufficient. Reconfirming with TOE may delayed surgical intervention and should be reserved for equivocal cases who remain well enough for the procedure. The requesting physician must be immediately contacted and surgery promptly organised to prevent death from rupture or valve insufficiency.

20 Answer C: 20–30 seconds

The left ventricular free wall is unlikely to have been involved in the patient's infarct hence the answer is when normal myocardium enhances.

21 Answer B: Attached by a thin stalk to the left side of the inter-atrial septum

Atrial myxomas are the most common primary cardiac tumour. They usually have non-specific symptoms, making early diagnosis a challenge. They are usually solitary (90%) and occur in the left atrial cavity (80%). Multifocal cardiac myxomas are associated with Carney's syndrome. Right-sided myxomas calcify more frequently than left-sided myxomas. The majority of atrial myxomas are attached to the inter-atrial septum via a small pedicle, but they occasionally arise from the wall of the atria or the valve surface.

22 Answer D: Aortic isthmus, just distal to the left subclavian artery

The ligamentum arteriosum fixes the thoracic aorta at the isthmus, making it most vulnerable to a tear in rapid deceleration and up to 90% of traumatic aortic tears occur at this site. Tears in the ascending aorta just distal to the aortic valve account for about 5%. Tears in the aortic arch and diaphragmatic hiatus constitute approximately 5%.

23 Answer C: Aortic arch

Syphilitic aneurysms occur in 10–12% of individuals with untreated syphilis and often develop 10–30 years after initial infection. The ascending aorta and arch are the most common sites and the aortic sinus the least. The majority of syphilitic aneurysms are saccular.

24 Answer D: Left atrial appendage

In the absence of a shunt, left-sided cardiac thrombus is most likely to be implicated in transient ischaemic events. Right-sided cardiac thrombi are likely to be filtered by the pulmonary circulation. The left atrial appendage is the most frequent site for a thrombus, especially in the context of known atrial fibrillation.

25 Answer A: Caffeine should be avoided as it can increase or decrease cardiac FDG uptake

Patients must be nil by mouth for four hours to maintain the blood glucose level, which will affect the rate of FDG 18 uptake by cells. High levels of glucose can compete with FDG uptake and degrade image quality and results, hence the glucose level should ideally be below 10 mg/L. Type 1 diabetic patients should be starved overnight and imaged first thing in the morning. If insulin is to be used, it should be administered at least one hour prior to FDG injection. Insulin increases FDG uptake in the heart, muscle and liver and can degrade image quality. Stimulants such as caffeine can have a variable effect on uptake. HbA1c has no effect on imaging.

26 Answer C: Cough fracture

This finding should be taken into context with the clinical history. If the patient had a history of malignancy, was older or had comorbidities, this finding should be viewed with more suspicion. Cough fractures can follow infection or inflammation or occur after fitting.

27 Answer C: High-sitting diaphragm causing artefact

Large patients often display artefact from the diaphragm and this should be checked while post processing the data. The inferior wall is usually supplied by the right coronary artery. The fact that both the rest and stress images are similar suggests that the findings are a result of artefact. Breast tissue in female patients can lead to similar findings.

28 Answer B: Ventilation/perfusion scan (V/Q)

D dimer should not be performed in high-risk patients such as this and imaging is the next step. Conventional angiography is the gold standard but is invasive and not available in most centres. The normal CXR and absence of concurrent disease leaves V/Q as the most appropriate test.

29 Answer E: Blalock-Taussig shunt

The Blalock-Taussig (B-T) shunt is an end-to-side anastomosis between the subclavian and pulmonary arteries performed for Tetralogy of Fallot and tricuspid atresia with pulmonary stenosis.

30 Answer B: Pulmonary hamartoma

Pulmonary hamartoma is the most common benign tumour of the lung. It is often asymptomatic and picked up incidentally on routine screening. They can be symptomatic if centrally located but the majority are peripheral. Popcorn calcification is visible in approximately 20% and fat density in half.

31 Answer E: Small intestine

32 Answer C: Fat embolism

In fat embolism, the perfusion defect is greater than the ventilation defect, resulting in a mismatched perfusion defect. With pulmonary infarction secondary to an embolus, there can be a matched ventilation/perfusion defect. Lung collapse, pleural effusion and emphysema result in mismatched ventilation defects.

33 Answer B: Right lower lobe

In Hydatid disease the parasite reaches the thorax via haematological spread from the liver. Lung lesions are usually single and located in the lower lobes or posterior mediastinum. The cyst can communicate with the bronchial tree. Complications include rupture and infection. Surgery may be required for excision.

34 Answer A: Pulmonary veins

Bronchopulmonary sequestration is a congenital malformation of a non-functioning lung segment that has no communication with the tracheobronchial tree and has a systemic blood supply. In intralobar sequestration, which is more common, aeration may occur via the pores of Kohn and venous drainage is via pulmonary veins to the left atrium. Venous drainage is via systemic veins in extralobar sequestration.

35 Answer A: Lung periphery

Rheumatoid nodules in the lungs are rare. They have the same composition as subcutaneous nodules and are most frequently located in the periphery. They do not calcify.

36 Answer B: Bronchial artery

Pulmonary carcinoid is a slow-growing low-grade malignant vascular tumour supplied by the bronchial circulation.

37 Answer B: Thymic cyst

Thymic hyperplasia and cysts may develop following radiotherapy to the thorax. Bronchogenic cysts are usually pericarinal in location. Half of these have water attenuation and the other half have higher attenuation due to the presence of mucous or milk of calcium contents. An air fluid level may be seen if it communicates with the airways. A pericardial cyst can be located in the mediastinal but it is very rare. Most pericardial cysts are located at the costophrenic angle, right more than left. They can change their shape and size with variation in respiration and position.

38 Answer A: Bronchopulmonary sequestration

This is a congenital anomaly resulting from independent development of part of the tracheobronchial tree, which may have a systemic arterial blood supply and classed into two types – intra and extralobar. The intralobar type is more common and classically presents in a young adult as recurrent pneumonia. They have a pulmonary venous drainage and are contained within the normal visceral pleura.

An extralobar sequestration has its own visceral pleura, drains into systemic veins and is usually asymptomatic.

39 Answer B: *Streptococcus pneumoniae*

Streptococcus pneumoniae is the commonest cause of all community-acquired bacterial pneumonias, and also the commonest cause of a round pneumonia, which are more common in children.

40 Answer B: Histoplasmosis

This is a typical history for histoplasmosis. It is usually symptomatic only in the very young and the older age group and more likely to be symptomatic in men. It is predominantly self-limiting and endemic to South America. The multiple punctate calcifications in the follow-up film with the history of self-limiting illness are also consistent with histoplasmosis, which is the commonest endemic mycosis. Tuberculosis is less likely to have the punctate calcifications a year later. Sarcoidosis usually presents in a younger age group.

41 Answer B: Langerhans cell histiocytosis (LCH)

Although the individual features can be seen in several of these conditions, the combination of the clinical history and radiological findings are most in keeping with LCH.

42 Answer C: Lymphangitis carcinomatosis

Pleural involvement in usual interstitial pneumonia (UIP) and sarcoidosis is unusual. In lymphoid interstitial pneumonia (LIP) there would almost certainly be centrilobular nodules and usually cysts. It would be unusual to see Kerley A and B lines in UIP, sarcoidosis or LIP. The normal heart size, nodular appearance to the septa and lymphadenopathy all make lymphangitis carcinomatosis more likely than LVF.

43 Answer D: Testis

Other primary malignancies causing calcification within metastases include breast, colon (mucinous adenocarcinoma), osteosarcoma and ovarian.

44 Answer B: Multiple small foci of calcification

Particularly adenocarcinomas that produce mucin can demonstrate multiple small foci of calcification. Popcorn calcification is diagnostic of a pulmonary hamartoma, complete or central calcification is seen in healed granulomas and concentric calcification is also indicative of granulomas.

45 Answer A: Prominent lymphadenopathy

Lymphadenopathy is a rare finding.

46 Answer C: Narrowing of the peripheral pulmonary vessels

The presence of enlarged pulmonary arteries on its own can be seen in acute and chronic thromboembolic disease, but narrowing of the peripheral vessels and often a mosaic attenuation pattern is much more suggestive of a chronic process.

47 Answer A: Pectus excavatum

The two findings are compatible with pectus excavatum as is a horizontal course of the posterior ribs and vertical course of the anterior ribs.

48 Answer B: Bronchial dilatation

The remaining findings are seen in bronchiolitis.

49 Answer D: α 1 antitrypsin deficiency

COPD is an unlikely diagnosis in this setting. CXR changes in Langerhans cell histiocytosis include reticulonodular opacification with relative basal sparing. Congenital lobar emphysema presents in infancy and most often affects a single lobe. LAM is seen in female patients. The findings of lower zone emphysema in a young patient are typical of α 1 antitrypsin deficiency.

50 Answer B: Schwannoma

The appearances are those of a posterior mediastinal mass. Thyroid/parathyroid masses, lymphoma and teratoma are most commonly seen within the anterior mediastinum. Although lymphoma remains a diagnostic possibility, a neurogenic tumour (e.g. schwannoma) is the most likely diagnosis in this case.

51 Answer A: Segmental perfusion defect much larger than an associated ventilation defect

Matched/Mismatched defects: A matched defect demonstrates both ventilation and perfusion abnormalities of similar size in the same region. A mismatched defect displays reduced perfusion in an area of normal ventilation, or a much larger perfusion defect than ventilation abnormality – typical of PE.

Segmental/Sub-segmental/Non-segmental defects: Occlusion of a segmental branch of the pulmonary artery will lead to a subpleural, wedge-shaped segmental perfusion defect – typical of PE. Sub-segmental perfusion defects are smaller than a whole segment. A non-segmental perfusion defect will not conform to segmental anatomy, that is will not appear wedge-shaped or sub-pleural.

52 Answer B: To accentuate differential lung attenuation caused by air trapping and obviate any gravitational (dependent) changes seen on the supine scan

Expiratory scanning is performed to accentuate the difference in attenuation between areas of trapped air and normal lung. Air trapping – caused by stenotic distal airways – is a feature of hypersensitivity pneumonitis, sarcoidosis and the pneumoconioses. Prone scanning can help differentiate between pathological areas of high attenuation seen in dependent locations on the supine scan from simple gravitational (dependent) change.

53 Answer B: Thyroid enlargement

The most common cause of a superior mediastinal mass is a goitre, followed by lymphadenopathy. Retrosternal goitres are seen to extend into the neck from the superior mediastinum and almost invariably displace or compress the trachea.

54 Answer E: Bronchogenic cyst

Bronchogenic cysts are budding abnormalities of the ventral diverticulum of the primitive foregut. They invariably contain mucoid material and are most commonly located in the mediastinum, although they can be seen within the lungs, where they predispose to infection. Tarlov cysts are dilated nerve root sleeves containing CSF.

55 Answer A: Acute interstitial pneumonitis (AIP)

AIP can be regarded as an idiopathic form of adult respiratory distress syndrome (ARDS) and is histologically (and clinically) distinct from the other interstitial pneumonias. The condition is usually preceded by a history of upper respiratory tract infection and the clinical picture is that of ARDS. Pathologically the findings are of diffuse alveolar damage, of which hyaline membrane formation is the characteristic feature.

56 Answer B: Drug-induced pulmonary damage

The most plausible explanation is drug-induced pulmonary damage from amiodarone (a commonly prescribed anti-arrhythmic medication). The picture is that of non-specific interstitial pneumonitis (NSIP) indicated by septal thickening and bilateral ground-glass change. Amiodarone deposition within the liver causes increased attenuation due to its high iodine content.

57 Answer D: Bilateral patchy segmental and lobar consolidation and ground-glass change

There are many causes of pulmonary haemorrhage including bleeding diathesis, trauma, haemorrhagic pneumonia and drug-related haemorrhage. Pulmonary haemorrhage in association with renal disease is common (e.g. Wegener's granulomatosis/Goodpasture's syndrome). The hallmark of diffuse pulmonary haemorrhage on imaging is multifocal consolidation and ground-glass change.

58 Answer B: Centrilobular emphysema in a predominantly mid and upper zone distribution and bronchial wall thickening

The clinical picture is that of chronic obstructive pulmonary disease (COPD), which is a smoking-related clinical entity comprising of chronic bronchitis and emphysema. Bronchitis manifests as bronchial wall thickening on CT. Emphysema describes abnormal permanent enlargement of airspaces distal to the terminal bronchiole caused by alveolar wall destruction. Different patterns of emphysema are described, but centrilobular and paraseptal emphysema are typically smoking related and preferentially affect the upper zones.

59 Answer D: Bilateral perihilar consolidation and ground-glass change

PCP can manifest in a number of ways. In 80% of cases there are diffuse, bilateral, symmetrical airspace infiltrates. Cysts (often perihilar) and diffuse interstitial infiltration can also occur. Often there is a combination of these forms. In 10% of cases no abnormality is seen on CXR. Pleural effusions and adenopathy have only rarely been described.

60 Answer C: A procedure where the patient's actions imply consent

Most radiological examinations involve minimal risk and the patient's actions are taken to represent implied consent. If there is any doubt as to the patient's understanding of the involved risk, formal verbal or written consent should be obtained. The GMC suggests that written consent should be taken in cases where: the treatment or procedure is complex and involves significant risk and/or side-effects, where providing clinical care is not the primary purpose of the investigation or procedure (in particular, where the examination or procedure is for non-therapeutic purposes), if the treatment is part of a research programme or if there may be significant consequences for the patient's employment, social or personal life. Written consent for some procedures is also required by the Mental Health Act and the Human Fertilisation and Embryology Act.

Royal College of Radiologists. *Standards for Patient Consent Particular to Radiology*. London: RCR; 2007. Available at: www.rcr.ac.uk/docs/radiology/pdf/CRpatientconsentweb.pdf (accessed 2 June 2009).

61 Answer A: Acute limb ischaemia

Indications for thrombolysis include: acute or acute-on-chronic ischaemia, graft thrombosis, thrombosed popliteal aneurysm and periprocedural thrombolysis.

62 Answer D: Narrow iliac arteries (<8 mm)

Although the exact measurements vary between EVAR systems, the principles are the same. Relative contraindications include: narrow (<8 mm) or angulated iliac arteries, short (<15 mm), angulated (>60 degrees) or tapering proximal neck or if the graft is likely to occlude visceral arteries. Graft technology is constantly evolving and new developments (e.g. fenestrated grafts) may overcome some of these issues.

63 Answer C: No immediate intervention: follow up but likely to be self-limiting

Type II endoleaks may cease if the aneurysm sac thromboses and the flow stops. If they persist, the aneurysmal sac may continue to expand.

64 Answer A: Right atrium

The chest radiograph findings suggest enlargement of the right atrium, which may be due to volume overload (ASD, AV canal, tricuspid incompetence, APVR) or pressure overload (tricuspid stenosis, right atrial mass).

65 Answer A: Aortic regurgitation

The cardiothoracic ratio is used as a guide to left ventricular dilatation. Often, the left ventricular volume has to increase by half to two-thirds before an increased ratio is easily appreciated. The ratio increases with expiration and supine positioning. In isolated mitral stenosis, there is dilatation of the left atrial appendage but the left ventricular size is often not enlarged.

66 Answer B: Transposition of the great vessels

Although Tetralogy of Fallot is the commonest cause in all age groups, this is the commonest cause of cyanosis in the neonatal period.

67 Answer D: Left upper lobe

A hyperlucent expanded lobe is seen (which may initially appear of soft tissue density due to retained fluid). The condition preferentially affects the left upper lobe (43%), right middle lobe (32%) and right upper lobe (20%). Two lobes are affected in 5%. Treatment is resection of the affected lobe.

68 Answer E: Passing inferiorly from the umbilicus to the pelvis then turning cranially to lie with the tip at T9

An umbilical artery catheter (UAC) should run into the pelvis via the umbilical artery to the iliac artery before turning superiorly to the aorta. An umbilical venous catheter will pass immediately superiorly. The tip of a UAC should not be positioned close to the origin of a major vessel T10-L3 due to risk of thrombosis.

69 Answer D: At the level of the thoracic inlet on the right posterolateral wall

Usually they occur between the cartilaginous and muscular portion of the wall and tend to be asymptomatic.

70 Answer C: Window width 700 HU, window level 100 HU

Musculoskeletal and trauma radiology

PAPER 1: ANSWERS AND EXPLANATIONS

1   Answer D: Achondroplasia

This syndrome has features affecting most body parts: skull (flat nasal bridge, broad mandible, etc.), chest (decreased AP distance, short anteriorly flared concave ribs), spine (anterior beak in lumbar spine, decreased vertebral body height, scoliosis), pelvis ('tombstone' iliac bones from squaring, 'champagne glass' pelvic inlet) and extremities ('trident' hand, short femoral necks, etc.). Homozygous achondroplasia is lethal. Roberts syndrome is a rare disorder displaying a phocomelia (similar to infants affected by thalidomide during pregnancy), and usually facial defects such as cleft lip and palate and malformed ears. Kniest syndrome is a newly described chondrodystrophy, the main features of which are flat, elongated and irregular vertebral bodies, dumbbell-shaped long bones and flattened, squared-off epiphyses of the hand. Pseudoachondroplastic patients have a normal face and head but display limb shortening, irregular epiphyses, scoliosis, coxa vara and marked shortening of bones in hands and feet.

2   Answer C: Amyloid arthropathy

Amyloid classically stains with Congo red and can be a primary or secondary process. Typical features include: bone pain, periarticular soft tissue swelling and carpal tunnel syndrome. Three patterns have been described: synovial articular pattern (amyloid arthropathy), diffuse marrow deposition and localised destructive lesion (amyloidoma, rarest form).

3   Answer E: Calvé-Kümmel-Verneuil disease

Also known as vertebral osteochondrosis or vertebra plana with appearances of a uniform collapse of a vertebral body into a flat, thin disc, with increased density of the vertebra. The intravertebral vacuum cleft sign is pathognomonic. Legg-Calvé-Perthe disease (coxa plana) is idiopathic femoral head avascular necrosis (males more commonly, peak at 4–8 years). Köhler disease is avascular necrosis of the tarsal scaphoid (males, 3–10 years). Kienböck's disease is AVN of the lunate, associated with negative ulnar variance in 75%. Freiberg disease is AVN of the metatarsal heads, age 10–18 years, females more often.

Theodorou DJ. Signs in imaging: the vacuum cleft phenomenon. *Radiology*. 2001; **221**(3): 787.

4 Answer C: Hyperparathyroidism

Calcium pyrophosphate dihydrate crystal deposition (CPPD) is frequently associated with osteoarthritis (OA), but is distinguished by the presence of chondrocalcinosis. This term describes the imaging appearances of the presence of calcium in cartilage; for example menisci, triangular fibrocartilage of wrist. Chondrocalcinosis may have other causes, therefore technically is not synonymous with CPPD. Common associations of CPPD are: hyperparathyroidism, hypothyroidism, haemochromatosis, hypomagnesaemia and haemosiderosis.

5 Answer A: Hypotelorism

Hypotelorism refers to an abnormally close distance between the eyes. Some of the features that occur with Trisomy 21 (Down syndrome) are: hypotelorism, atlantoaxial subluxation, flattening of the acetabular roof, metaphyseal flaring and anterior scalloping of the vertebral bodies. Consider abnormalities in the following categories: skull, axial skeleton, chest, pelvis, extremities and gastrointestinal.

6 Answer A: 4 (cases per million per year)

The incidence is a measure of the number of new cases in a period of time. The prevalence is the total number of cases present in the population.

7 Answer C: Linear symmetrical cortical uptake seen most avidly along the posterior aspects of the tibiae

Patchy uptake in shafts is more likely to indicate stress fracture, which may present in a similar fashion. The uptake in shin splints is usually diagnostic, but lateral views of the lower limbs are necessary to demonstrate the uptake along the posterior cortices. The hot patella sign is non-specific but not associated with the diagnosis of shin splints.

8 Answer D: Monostotic

Fibrous dysplasia is a skeletal developmental anomaly of bone forming mesenchyme, which manifests as a defect in osteoblastic differentiation and maturation. Almost any bone can be affected. Monostotic is found in 70–80%. Polyostotic is found in 20–30% and can be associated with endocrine dysfunction and café au lait spots in 10%. Craniofacial is rarer (10–25% of monostotic, 50% of polyostotic). The familial form is rare.

9 Answer C: Likely aggressive processes

Periosteum is composed of two layers, outer fibrous and inner cellular, which has potential for osteoblastic potential. It is more active in childhood and therefore is visualised earlier in children. Periosteal reaction represents either new bone formation or periosteal elevation. The different types of periosteal reaction are: lamellated, solid, speculated, sunburst or hair on end, Codman's triangle. Tumours presenting with speculated, sunburst, disorganised periosteal reaction or Codman's triangle are likely to represent aggressive processes.

Wenaden A, Szyszko T. Imaging of periosteal reactions associated with focal lesions of bone. *Clin Radiol.* 2005; **60**(4): 439–56.

10 Answer C: Scoliosis

Skeletal abnormalities occur in 25–40% of cases of NF1 and the most common skeletal abnormality is scoliosis. These abnormalities are either due to pressure effects from adjacent neurofibromas or underlying mesenchymal abnormality. Erosion by neurofibromas of the intercostal nerves, leads to loss of bone of the superior and inferior aspects of the ribs and the abnormality known as 'ribbon ribs'. Other abnormalities include: bowing of bone, pseudoarthrosis and cystic osteolytic lesions. The vertebrae demonstrate posterior scalloping and enlargement of the intervertebral foraminae, secondary to neurofibromas of the nerve roots.

Hillier JC, Moskovic E. The soft-tissue manifestations of neurofibromatosis type 1. *Clin Radiol.* 2005; **60**(9): 960–7.

11 Answer A: A 'squared' patella

Haemophilia is an X-linked condition, which affects males. Haemophilic arthropathy is caused by repeated bleeding into the joint, leading to pannus formation, which erodes cartilage and leads to loss of the subchondral bone plate and formation of subarticular cysts. Patients present in the first or second decade with a tense, red, warm joint and decreased range of movement. There is associated fever and elevated white count. On MR, low signal is returned from the hypertrophied synovium due to magnetic susceptibility of haemosiderin.

12 Answer B: Dolichocephaly (scaphocephaly)

Marfan syndrome is a connective tissue disorder of a mutation in the fibrillin-1 gene. It affects various systems: musculoskeletal, ocular, cardiovascular (in 60–98%), pulmonary and abdominal. The main musculoskeletal areas involved are: skull, hands, feet, spine and joints, with arachnodactyly, dolichocephaly, hallux valgus, scoliosis. Arachnodactyly is elongation of the phalanges and metacarpals. Dolichocephaly is where the head is disproportionately long and narrow. The fifth finger demonstrates a flexion deformity.

Ha HI, Seo JB, Lee SH, *et al.* Imaging of Marfan syndrome: multisystemic manifestations. *RadioGraphics.* 2007; **27**(4): 989–1004.

13 Answer A: Bilateral posterior iliac horns

Nail-patella syndrome is a rare autosomal dominant disorder with features of symmetrical meso- and ectodermal abnormalities. The aetiology is possibly a defect in collagen metabolism. It generally becomes apparent in second and third decades with hypoplasia or absence of thumb and index fingernails, an abnormal gait and renal dysfunction. The diagnostic feature radiographically is bilateral posterior iliac horns, which are present in 80%.

14 Answer B: No need for specific treatment, spontaneous resolution is likely

Non-ossifying fibromas are also known as fibroxanthoma, fibrous medullary defect and several other synonyms. They are found in up to 40% of children less than two years old. They are generally painless and found in shafts of long bones, mostly lower limb particularly around the knee. They tend to be eccentric within the metaphysis, mostly in the medulla. Multiple lesions have several associations; Neurofibromatosis, fibrous dysplasia, Jaffe-Campanacci syndrome. They tend to be aligned along the axis of the long bone and measure around 2 cm in length. If they are more than 3.3 cm and occupy more than half of the bone diameter, they should be observed. Mostly, these lesions spontaneously resolve.

15 Answer A: Osseous expansion

Paget's is a multifocal skeletal process, which results from disordered and excessive bone remodelling. It has several stages: active, osteolytic phase, middle, mixed phase and an inactive, quiescent late phase. Radiography alone is only 13–74% sensitive. Scintigraphy and radiography are 60% sensitive. Bone scan alone is over 90% sensitive. Commonly affected areas are: skull, long bones, ribs, pelvis and spine. The key features are osseous expansion with thickening of the cortex and coarsening of the trabecular pattern.

16 Answer B: Osteopetrosis

Osteopetrosis is also known as marble bone disease and is a rare disease of abnormal osteoclast activity where there is failure of resorption and remodelling, which leads to sclerotic, thick bone, which is weak and brittle. The types include: infantile autosomal recessive (is either fatal in utero or life expectancy is up to middle age), benign adult autosomal dominant, phenotypes 1 and 2 (normal life expectancy). The metaphyseal striations are longitudinal.

17 Answer E: Joint effusion

The knee is the most common location for PVNS. The soft tissues appear dense due to haemosiderin deposits and there are multiple sites of cyst-like radiolucent defects due to bone invasion. There is not usually any evidence of calcification, osteoporosis and joint space narrowing until later on. There is low signal on all sequences due to the presence of haemosiderin. Other features include: knee joint effusion on plain films, scalloping of pre-femoral fat pad, soft-tissue mass around joint, no joint space narrowing.

18 Answer B: Caplan's syndrome

Caplan's syndrome is a hyperimmune reactivity to silica inhalation with rapidly developing pulmonary nodules. Felty's syndrome is RA plus splenomegaly and osteopenia. Panner's disease is osteonecrosis of the capitellum.

19 Answer A: Reticulated trabecular pattern

Osseous involvement in sarcoid is uncommon, being reported in 6–20% of cases, and tends to affect the small bones of the hands and feet. The key features are a reticulated trabecular pattern, cyst-like lesions and destruction of the terminal phalanges. Other bony lesions are diffuse sclerosis of vertebral bodies and osteo-lytic changes in the skull.

20 Answer D: Periosteal reaction

Periosteal reaction is a frequent finding in psoriatic arthritis. Twenty per cent of patients with psoriasis develop psoriatic arthropathy which is classified into true psoriatic, resembling rheumatoid and concomitant rheumatoid and psori-atic type. The onset of arthritis often precedes the skin rash. The distribution is variable and asymmetrical, affecting hand and foot and axial skeleton. Features include 'pencil in cup' deformity, ivory phalanx, squaring of vertebrae and atlan-toaxial subluxation.

21 Answer A: Acute fracture

All the other answers are for causes of an abnormal bone scan with no findings (or minimal changes) on plain radiography. Causes of a positive radiograph with a normal bone scan are: metabolically inactive benign conditions (bone cysts/ bone island/exostoses), recent fractures (less than 48 hours), multiple myeloma, osteoporosis, and rarely metastases if there is no osteoblastic activity.

22 Answer A: Intra-articular loose body

23 Answer D: One-shot IVU following intravenous contrast medium administra-tion

In an unstable patient, there is no time for a CT scan, and a 'one-shot' IVU would be the simplest and most effective study prior to potential surgery. CT remains the investigation of choice in any blunt abdominal trauma in a stable patient.

24 Answer B: Neurofibromatosis type 1

These features are typical of the appearance of the spine. In NF1 the muscu-loskeletal manifestations tend to predominate.

25 Answer C: Comminuted calcaneal fractures

Predictable patterns of injury after a fall from a height include: calcaneal, pelvic and thoraco-lumbar spine fractures. A Maisonneuve fracture is a proximal fibular fracture commonly associated with a medial malleolar avulsion fracture.

26 Answer D: Contrast-enhanced CT chest

A widened mediastinum is sensitive, but not specific for blunt aortic injury. Accordingly, contrast-enhanced CT (or trans-oesophageal echocardiography) should be performed to exclude aortic injury.

27 Answer A: Sacrum

Osteoporotic sacral insufficiency fractures have a classical H-shaped configuration.

28 Answer D: Lisfranc fracture-dislocation

A fracture of the first or second metatarsal in conjunction with a dislocation of the tarso-metatarsal articulation is termed a Lisfranc fracture-dislocation. Such injuries usually require a significant force. A fracture of the medial malleolus usually occurs as a result of an inversion injury. A fracture of the proximal fibula (with disruption of the proximal talofibular syndesmosis) in conjunction with a fracture of the medial malleolus is termed a Maisonneuve fracture. Diabetics are at risk of peripheral neuropathy and subsequent injury due to lack of sensation and the commonest cause of a Charcot joint in the Western world is diabetes.

29 Answer B: Torn ligament between the second metatarsal and medial cuneiform

An injury to the Lisfranc joint most commonly occurs at the joint involving the first and second metatarsals and the medial cuneiform. The Lisfranc ligament is the only ligament connecting the second metatarsal to the medial cuneiform and may be torn with a Lisfranc injury. While transverse ligaments connect the bases of the lateral four metatarsals, no transverse ligament exists between the first and second metatarsal bases. The joint capsule and Lisfranc ligament form the only minimal support on the dorsal surface of the Lisfranc joint. As many as 20% of Lisfranc joint injuries are missed on initial anteroposterior and oblique radiographs.

30 Answer E: No further imaging – rest and occupational modification alone are adequate

The history is highly suggestive of pre-patellar bursitis. Hence no further imaging is required. Removal of provocative factors and rest are normally adequate. Use of kneepads may also be of benefit. Complications such as secondary infection may necessitate antibiotic therapy.

31 Answer A: Mandibular condyle

The site of mandibular fractures in order of frequency: condyle (30%), angle (25%), symphysis/parasymphysis (22%), body (16%), dentoalveolar ligament (3%), ramus (2%), coronoid process (1%).

32 Answer B: Uncemented hemi-arthroplasty

The treatment of choice for an intra-capsular (subcapital) femoral neck fracture in an elderly patient is hemi-arthroplasty. In a younger patient group, cannulated screws could be considered. Dynamic hip screws are indicated for extra-capsular fractures where there is little risk of avascular necrosis from femoral head devascularisation.

33 Answer E: Triquetral

Triquetral fractures are common although easily missed on standard frontal projections. On a lateral projection an avulsed flake of bone lying posterior to the triquetral is typical. The usual mechanism of injury is falling onto an outstretched hand in ulnar deviation. A less common mechanism of triquetral fracture is a direct blow to the dorsum of the hand, which would usually be accompanied by other carpal fractures as a greater force is required. A fall onto an outstretched hand more commonly causes a scaphoid fracture although this is more likely in radial rather than ulnar deviation.

34 Answer D: Rupture of ulnar collateral ligament

Chronic injury of this ligament is termed 'gamekeeper's thumb' but the acute form is now much more common and is termed 'skier's thumb' due to acute forceful abduction of the thumb usually when trapped in a ski pole. The ulnar collateral ligament originates from the first metacarpal head and may avulse a small fragment of bone from its proximal phalangeal insertion. Subluxation, but not usually frank dislocation, of this joint is seen and prompt consideration of surgical repair is indicated to prevent prolonged pain and functional impairment.

35 Answer C: Bilateral facet dislocation

This injury is inherently unstable, in contrast to unilateral facet dislocation. Severe flexion forces in combination with distraction result in complete disruption of the facet joints and displacement of the vertebral body by at least 50% relative to the one below it. A significant number are associated with traumatic disc herniation. Initial closed reduction and traction is required, but should be done judiciously as it is possible for a disc herniation to retropulse into the cervical canal.

36 Answer A: Osteoblastoma

Osteoblastomas are clinically and histologically similar to osteoid osteoma with a nidus as a characteristic feature. Enchondromas often have multiple lytic lesions, but there is no nidus. A giant cell tumour is a trabeculated bone lesion. Fibrous dysplasia would be a possibility but the description is classical for an osteoblastoma and fibrous dysplasia more frequently affects the proximal femur.

37 Answer B: Haemangioma

Haemangiomas are confined to trabecular bone. Their characteristic appearance is due to resorption of trabeculae by enlarged vascular channels and thickening of the remaining trabeculae.

38 Answer C: Chondroblastoma

Chondroblastomas usually occur from 5–20 years and are almost exclusively epiphyseal. Osteosarcomas and non-ossifying fibromas are usually metaphyseal. Lymphoma and Ewing sarcomas are usually diaphyseal.

39 Answer A: To biopsy a deep lesion

Although more expensive, introducer-sheathed biopsy needles have the advantage of allowing deeper biopsies to be taken. They are often used for smaller, more difficult to target biopsies. Smaller specimens are taken with introducer-sheathed needles.

40 Answer C: Lymphoma

Lymphoma of bone is more commonly non-Hodgkin's lymphoma and is predominantly diaphyseal. None of the other lesions are classically diaphyseal nor would they explain his constitutional symptoms.

41 Answer A: Paget's disease

A flame-shaped lucency and bone expansion with cortical thickening are typical features of Paget's disease. An aneurysmal bone cyst would have thin, intact cortex and tends to affect the metaphysis. Non-ossifying fibromas usually present in children.

42 Answer E: Giant cell tumour

Giant cell tumours are seen in skeletally mature patients. They are epiphyseal/metaphyseal, most common in the distal femur and do not cause surrounding sclerosis. Desmoplastic fibromas are osteolytic and metaphyseal but usually have well-defined sclerotic margins. Aneurysmal bone cysts do occur in this age but are metaphyseal and one would expect to see fluid levels within the cystic spaces on MRI. Metastatic breast deposits are generally diaphyseal and rare in this age group. Enchondromas are diaphyseal and have matrix mineralisation.

43 Answer A: Wide resection and reconstruction with allograft

Allograft resection is the treatment of choice for a large giant cell tumour causing destruction. A wide resection is preferred as a marginal resection is associated with a high recurrence rate. Chemotherapy has no role in the management of this tumour.

44 Answer C: Osteosarcoma

Osteosarcoma is a high-grade intramedullary tumour. It has high signal on T2W MRI due to replacement of the normal bone marrow and foci of high signal on T1W MRI because of central haemorrhage. An osteoid osteoma would not have significant periosteal reaction. Osteochondroma is painless with no periosteal reaction. Chondromyxoid fibroma occurs in the third or fourth decade. It is a lucent lesion with a sclerotic rim. Chondrosarcoma is unlikely in this age group, usually present over 40 years of age.

45 Answer B: Chondroblastoma

Chondroblastoma typically occur in this age group and are epiphyseal, well-defined lucencies with a thin sclerotic rim. Osteosarcoma, fibrosarcoma and clear cell chondrosarcoma would be expected to have more aggressive features. Osteomas occur in the elderly population and tend to be sclerotic.

46 Answer A: Osteosarcoma

Osteosarcomas are the most common and aggressive primary bone tumours. Despite the potential of arising in any bone, the majority arise in the metaphyseal growth plates of long bones. Other sites are the pelvis and jaw. The peak incidence is in the second and third decades but there is a second peak in the seventh and eighth decades, chiefly as a result of malignant transformation in Paget's disease.

47 Answer E: Chondromyxoid fibroma

The proximal tibial metaphysis is a classic location for a chondromyxoid fibroma which is always benign, hence there is a lack of periosteal reaction and soft-tissue involvement. Aneurysmal bone cysts do occur in the metaphysis; usually a thinned cortex and fluid-fluid levels are visible.

48 Answer C: Percutaneous radiofrequency ablation

Percutaneous RFA is the treatment of choice for osteoid osteoma and primary success rates of up to 90% are reported. With secondary recurrence, repeat RFA leads to an even higher success rate approaching 100%. Chemotherapy and irradiation are not indicated in the treatment of these tumours. Resection, curettage, cryotherapy, bone grafting and prosthetic replacement are invasive with a greater risk of incomplete excision.

49 Answer A: Fibrous dysplasia

The popcorn-shaped calcifications are cartilage-producing nodules, which are typical of fibrous dysplasia.

50 Answer C: *Staphylococcus aureus*

Some series suggest that *Salmonella* is the most likely cause but others have found that *Staphylococcus* is the commonest cause in this population.

51 Answer D: Simple bone cyst

Simple bone cysts often have prominent fluid levels. They commonly present in the second decade and are slightly expansile. Aneurysmal bone cysts have more marked expansion with fluid-fluid levels and tend to occur in an older age group. Fibrous dysplasia is unlikely as it is not an entirely lytic lesion. Giant cell tumour is lytic but often has septations. With brown tumours there is osteoclastic activity due to hyperparathyroidism, so there would usually be osteopenia.

52 Answer A: Ewing sarcoma

With Ewing sarcoma 'onion skinning' reflects the periodic activity of the sarcoma interspersed with quiescent periods. Brodie's abscess is high on the differential given the systemic upset, but usually has a lytic area with surrounding sclerosis.

Trauma is not likely due to the insidious onset. Neuroblastoma typically occurs under the age of five.

53 Answer D: Sacrum

When Ewing's affects the spine the sacrum is most commonly affected, followed by the lumbar, thoracic and cervical regions in that order.

54 Answer E: Thinned cortex with mild expansion

Simple bone cysts are fluid-filled lesions of unknown aetiology. They are most common in males in the first two decades of life and are metaphyseal lesions which migrate into the diaphysis over time. They may have thin internal septae and a thin sclerotic rim is often present.

55 Answer D: Non-Hodgkin's lymphoma

It is very rare for Hodgkin's disease to present in bone and most intraosseous lymphomas are of the non-Hodgkin's type.

56 Answer C: Osteosarcoma

Osteosarcoma is an aggressive lesion that can be mixed lytic/sclerotic in appearance and is common at this age and site. Granulocytic sarcoma occurs in patients with leukaemia or other myeloproliferative disorder but is rarely sclerotic. Ewing sarcoma has a moth-eaten appearance and is usually lytic. Aneurysmal bone cysts are not aggressive. Osteoid osteoma has a nidus and no bony destruction.

57 Answer B: Osteochondroma

Diaphyseal aclasis is the condition of multiple hereditary osteochondromas. It is an autosomal dominant disorder in which multiple osteochondromas are seen throughout the skeleton, preferentially affecting the long bones. It is associated with short stature and asymmetrical growth leading to deformities.

58 Answer C: Aneurysmal bone cyst

An aneurysmal bone cyst is very vascular hence exhibits increased uptake in the blood-pool phase. A simple bone cyst has no uptake. An enostosis has no uptake.

59 Answer E: Sclerotic osteosarcoma

Ivory vertebrae occur due to an increase in opacity of a vertebral body while retaining its size and contours. The differential also includes osteoblastic metastases with sclerotic response, Paget's disease, osteopetrosis, fluorosis, lymphoma and myelosclerosis. Osteomyelitis does produce sclerosis in vertebrae, but it rarely affects a single vertebra and one would expect erosive change at the endplates.

60 Answer B: Cervical spine

Almost two-thirds occur in the cervical spinal cord with one-third of these showing extension to the thoracic cord. They usually extend over multiple segments (three or four on average).

61 Answer E: Geographic bone destruction with a prominent sclerotic rim

No periosteal reaction is present unless there is a fracture. Internal septation is common and there is often thinning of the overlying cortex.

62 Answer B: 10–20 years

Chondroblastomas present as a well-defined lucency usually in the femur, proximal humerus or proximal tibia. Internal calcification is visible in 60% and there is usually florid marrow oedema on MRI.

63 Answer E: Pathologic fracture

Malignant degeneration is rare, particularly in solitary peripheral lesions. It is more common with multiple lesions and in more central lesions. Unless it occurs no systemic symptoms occur.

64 Answer E: Vertebral body

Usually in upper lumbar/lower thoracic spine. Rarely may bulge posterior cortex or extend into spinal canal leading to cord compression.

65 Answer D: 1 Male: 2 Female

Most bone tumours either have an even sex distribution or are more common in men except Ewing's, aneurismal bone cysts, haemangiomas and giant cell tumours.

66 Answer D: Well-defined cortical lesion with no periosteal reaction

Brown tumours occur in hyperparathyroidism and are most common in the primary form. They are also known as osteoclastomas due to parathyroid hormone-stimulated osteoclastic activity. These tumours are eccentric/cortical and are usually solitary.

67 Answer C: Palmoplantar pustulosis

The patient has SAPHO syndrome (synovitis, acne, palmoplantar pustulosis, hyperostosis and osteitis).

68 Answer C: Neurofibromatosis

Other possibilities are fibrous dysplasia or osteogenesis imperfecta. Non-union could give this appearance but it is unlikely given the history.

69 Answer E: Autosomal dominant

The patient has cleidocranial dysostosis.

70 Answer A: No increased risk

The patient has osteopoikilosis, which is not premalignant or associated with other malignancies. Gardner's syndrome is a familial polyposis syndrome associated with bone islands, but the usual finding is of fewer larger bone islands.

Musculoskeletal and trauma radiology

PAPER 2: ANSWERS AND EXPLANATIONS

1 Answer A: Heel pad thickness >25 mm

The underlying condition is acromegaly, indicated by the bitemporal hemianopia and excess growth hormone secretion. Normal heel pad thickness is <21 mm. Although heel pad thickness is not limited to acromegaly, it is the only condition in the list that is caused by a pituitary tumour. The list can be remembered by 'MAD COP' = Myxoedema, Acromegaly, Dilantin (phenytoin) therapy, Callus, Obesity, Peripheral oedema.

2 Answer B: Sclerosis and flattening of the metatarsal head

The scenario described is of Freiberg disease, osteochondrosis of the head of the second (third and fourth) metatarsal heads in 10–18 year olds, usually women (M:F 1:3). Clinically they present with metatarsalgia, swelling and tenderness. Early and late features are seen. Early on, flattening and cystic lesions of the metatarsal head are seen, with widening of the metatarsophalangeal joint. Late features include: an osteochondral fragment, sclerosis and flattening of the bone and increased cortical thickening.

3 Answer E: Spontaneous osteonecrosis of the knee (SONK)

This condition is most common in the seventh decade (range of 13–83 years) and occurs with acute pain. It is thought to be associated with a meniscal tear and microfractures (secondary to trauma), but there are multiple predisposing causes. An early bone scan (<5 weeks) would show pathology. Findings on delayed films include:

- flattening of the weight-bearing area of the medial femoral condyle;
- a radiolucent focus in the subchondral bone;
- later, subchondral fracture and periosteal reaction, which can lead to osteoarthritis in around half.

Panner's disease is osteonecrosis of the capitellum. The history is too acute for metastases or lymphoma. A benign cortical defect is more likely in first and second decades and is usually asymptomatic.

4   Answer A: Increased signal intensity on T2WI

The pathogenesis of carpal tunnel is probably one of ischaemia with venous congestion and nerve oedema from anoxia of the capillaries followed by impairment of venous and arterial blood supply. There are multiple causes for carpal tunnel syndrome including physiological states such as pregnancy. Other radiological features include: 'pseudoneuroma' of median nerve, swelling of nerve within carpal tunnel, volar bowing of flexor retinaculum, tenosynovitis of tendon sheaths, enhancement of the median nerve due to oedema or alternatively no enhancement due to ischaemia from holding the wrist in a fixed flexed/extended position.

5   Answer A: Aortography

Aortography is contraindicated because of the complications of aortic rupture and haematoma. Ehlers-Danlos is an autosomal disease of connective tissue due to altered collagen synthesis. There are 10 types, mostly in males. Features affect the following systems: soft tissues, skeleton, chest, arteries and GI tract.

6   Answer C: Weight-bearing load area of knee producing uptake

Bone scan appearances of knee replacements can take up to 18 months to normalise, as it is such a dynamic, weight-bearing joint. Loosening should be correlated with plain film findings such as adjacent bone lucency. The presence of normal inflammatory markers is reassuring, but subclinical infection should be considered with increased uptake in dynamic imaging. The hips and spine should be routinely imaged in lower limb pain to exclude referred pain. Load bearing changes on the medial aspect of the tibial plateau are not specific to joint replacements and in this case is the most likely cause of the pain.

7   Answer B: Monostotic Paget's disease

These are typical appearances but radiological correlation should be performed.

8   Answer E: Periosteal new bone formation

A soft-tissue ganglion is a cystic tumour-like lesion usually attached to a tendon sheath. It can present with a painful or a painless lump, most commonly over the hand, wrist or foot. The T1-weighted imaging characteristics are typically low to intermediate signal. Other features include: communication with joint, high signal on T2, internal septations, periosteal new bone formation. The natural history is spontaneous resolution although steroid injections may improve symptoms. Other types of ganglion include intraosseous and periosteal.

9   Answer C: Blurring of the periarticular fat planes is common

Septic arthritis usually occurs in hip, knee, shoulder, elbow and ankle. *Staphylococcus aureus*, followed by group A *Streptococcus*, are the most common causes. Other radiographic features include periarticular soft-tissue swelling, an effusion, periarticular osteopenia and, later, joint space narrowing. Ultrasound may help identify septic arthritis before cartilage lysis occurs. The hallmark is joint effusion in a patient with signs of a joint infection.

Chau CL, Griffith JF. Musculoskeletal infections: ultrasound appearances. *Clin Radiol.* 2005; **60**(2): 149–59.

10 Answer E: Metacarpophalangeal joints of index and middle fingers

This classical distribution is distinctive although not every case will show the classical findings.

11 Answer A: Jaccoud's arthropathy

This primarily affects the hands and occasionally the hallux. Radiographic features include muscular atrophy, periarticular swelling of the small joints of hands and feet, ulnar deviation and flexion of the MCP joints most marked in fourth and fifth finger without joint narrowing or erosion.

12 Answer E: Myositis ossificans

This is also known as heterotopic ossification, pseudomalignant tumour of soft tissue and extraosseous localised non-neoplastic bone and cartilage formation. It is a benign solitary self-limiting ossifying soft tissue mass typically occurring within skeletal muscle. Direct trauma is the cause in 75%. The pathology is of a lesion surrounded by compressed fibrous connective tissue and surrounded by atrophic skeletal muscle. The symptoms include pain, tenderness and soft-tissue mass. It has a progressive natural history where it resolves spontaneously, which is reflected in its plain film and MR characteristics.

13 Answer A: Charcot-Marie-Tooth

Neuropathic osteoarthropathy is a traumatic arthritis associated with loss of sensation and proprioception of the affected limb. The causes can be congenital (Charcot-Marie-Tooth, Ehlers-Danlos), acquired (central/peripheral neuropathy, neurosyphilis, diabetes mellitus) or iatrogenic. Iatrogenic causes include: prolonged use of systemic or intra-articular steroids, and prolonged use of pain relieving drugs.

14 Answer B: Hair-on-end appearance of skull

Iron deficiency anaemia is caused by deficient iron stores at birth, dietary deficiency or excess blood loss for example, due to menstruation or from the gastrointestinal tract. Features are: widening of diploe, hair-on-end appearance of skull, osteoporosis in long bones and absence of facial bone involvement. Biconcave vertebrae occur in sickle cell anaemia.

15 Answer C: Hydrocephalus

(Secondary to basilar impression) The four main categories for complications of Paget's disease are: associated neoplasia, insufficiency fractures, neurologic entrapment, and early onset osteoarthritis.

Neoplasia includes sarcomatous transformation, multicentric giant cell tumour or lymphoma. Banana fractures are tiny horizontal 'Looser lines' on convex surfaces of lower extremity long bones. Other insufficiency fractures include vertebral compression fractures. Neurologic complications involve either basilar impression leading to hydrocephalus and brainstem compression, or spinal stenosis.

16 Answer E: Tapered margin of distal clavicle

Rheumatoid arthritis (RA) is a connective disease with associated immune complex deposition. There are early and late signs of the disease. RA affects hand and wrist, cervical spine, ribs, shoulder, hips, knee and feet. The main features are: erosions, loss of joint space, subchondral sclerosis. Other features include: osteoporosis, scalloped erosion on undersurface of clavicle, tapered margin of distal clavicle.

17 Answer D: Slipped upper femoral epiphysis (SUFE)

SUFE typically occurs in overweight boys (M:F 3:1, mean age 13 in boys, 11 in girls). There are many causes and associations. Patients may present with hip or knee pain or a limp. It occurs bilaterally in less than one-third. It is graded on the extent of the femoral head slip.

18 Answer C: Psoriatic arthritis

Other causes are juvenile rheumatoid arthritis, infectious arthritis and Reiter's syndrome.

19 Answer B: Calcaneonavicular

Calcaneonavicular and talocalcaneal coalitions each account for approximately 45%.

20 Answer C: Madelung's deformity

Turner's syndrome is due to an X0 genotype and patients are usually of short stature. Associated abnormalities include: coarctation, aortic stenosis, horseshoe kidneys, a shield-shaped chest, squared lumbar vertebrae and thinned ribs.

Madelung's deformity is due to abnormal growth at the distal radial physis leading to a volar and ulnar tilt to the distal radius with overgrowth of the ulna. It is associated with Turner's syndrome, dyschondrosteosis and diaphyseal aclasis but may also be post-traumatic or post-infective.

21 Answer B: Dental disease

A radiotherapy field is a photopenic area (along with internal or external artefacts, avascular lesions, multiple myeloma, haemangioma and advance carcinoma). Increased uptake can be pathological of physiological. Pathological factors include: metastatic disease, joint disease, traumatic or stress fracture, postoperatively, Paget's, disseminated secondary disease, metabolic bone disease and dental infection. Physiological factors include: artefacts, age factors, soft-tissue uptake.

22   Answer D: Just distal to left subclavian artery

Rapid deceleration is the usual cause of aortic rupture and this usually occurs just distal to the origin of the great vessels.

23   Answer D: 4 minutes

The aim is to acquire the images once contrast has reached the bladder and of the options available 4 minutes is the best choice.

24   Answer C: It controls lateral meniscal displacement

The popliteus muscle unlocks the knee from a position of full extension by internally rotating the tibia. It therefore initiates knee flexion. It limits posterior tibial translation and prevents excessive external rotation and varus rotation of the tibia during knee flexion. It is part of the structures of the posterolateral corner of the knee.

   Wheeler LD. Isolated popliteus tendon avulsion in skeletally immature patients. *Clin Radiol*. 2008; **63**(7): 824–8.

25   Answer E: CT head and cervical spine

Multidetector CT with coronal and sagittal reformatting is now commonplace and the gold standard for cervical spine trauma.

26   Answer A: Fracture of the shaft of the fifth metacarpal

This is often termed a 'boxer's fracture'. A Bennett's fracture is an intra-articular fracture-dislocation of the base of the thumb metacarpal and Rolando fractures are intra-articular comminuted fractures of the base of the thumb metacarpal.

27   Answer E: Tibialis posterior

Spontaneous tibialis posterior rupture tends to occur in those with underlying pathology, especially rheumatoid arthritis. The typical presentation is in a woman of 40–60 years and the presenting signs and symptoms are pain, difficulty walking, and swelling along the medial malleolus and the arch of the foot. Traumatic rupture is more common in a younger age group and is not normally secondary to another pathology.

28   Answer C: A bi-convex collection of high density adjacent to a linear lucency in the skull vault

The history is classical for an extra-dural haematoma in which a lucent interval may precede rapid deterioration and prompt neurosurgical evacuation is curative. The haemorrhage is frequently secondary to middle meningeal artery rupture, classically associated with a fracture at the pterion. Small high-attenuation foci (contusions) would be unlikely with the given history and are generally managed conservatively. A crescentic mixed-attenuation collection would be more likely to represent an organising subdural haematoma.

29 Answer C: Intraperitoneal free fluid

In a recent study, intraperitoneal free fluid had 100% sensitivity for surgically important bowel or mesenteric injury in the context of blunt abdominal trauma. (although the specificity was only 26% in this context). Other signs are much less sensitive but are much more specific, e.g. abrupt mesenteric vessel termination (sensitivity 45%, specificity 93%) or mesenteric vessel beading (sensitivity 50%, specificity 95%).

Atri M, Hanson JM, Grinblat L, *et al*. Surgically important bowel and/or mesenteric injury in blunt trauma: accuracy of multidetector CT for evaluation. *Radiology*. 2008; **249**(2): 524–33.

30 Answer D: Clay-shoveller's fracture

A clay shoveller's fracture is a stable fracture of a lower cervical vertebra spinous process, usually C7. The mechanism is sudden flexion of the neck combined with a heavy upper body and lower neck muscular contraction. This causes avulsion of the spinous process by the supraspinous ligament. A similar fracture may also occur with direct blows to the spinous process or with occipital trauma causing forced flexion of the neck. The remaining fractures are all potentially unstable.

31 Answer A: MCL rupture due to valgus stress

Isolated medial collateral ligament (MCL) injuries usually result from a valgus stress without a rotary component. They are more commonly associated with other injuries (e.g. ACL and medial meniscal tears) but isolated MCL tears are sometimes seen.

32 Answer A: Vertebral body

The most common site for metastatic involvement is the anterior aspect of the vertebral body. Increased uptake in the posterior elements and especially facet joints is more suggestive of degenerative change.

33 Answer E: Discontinuity at musculotendinous junction of adductor longus muscle

Acute adductor strain is caused by forceful adduction of the thigh during an abduction movement. This sudden change in direction requires powerful contraction of the adductor muscles, which may tear to varying degrees depending on the adequacy of prior stretching and the force of the movement. Unless there is a complete tear, loss of function will not result, though there may be pain, swelling and ecchymoses on the anteromedial aspect of the thigh. Ultrasound may confirm the presence of a tear, which is often seen at the musculotendinous junction.

34 Answer D: Pilon fracture

A high-energy impact where the talus is driven into the tibia can result in a Pilon fracture. Alternatively, a fall from a height may lead to another pattern of injuries such as a comminuted fracture of the calcaneum or fractures of the pelvis or lumbar spine. A multiplanar CT examination is useful for operative planning to show the extent of the fracture.

35 Answer A: Zygomatic arch fracture

Zygomatic arch fractures usually result from a direct blow to the side of the face and the classical presentation is with flattening of the cheek and an inability to open the mouth due to impingement of the fracture fragment upon the coronoid process of the mandible or the temporalis muscle. Multiplanar CT is usually indicated although the best radiographic view is the SMV projection if CT is not available.

36 Answer D: Aneurysmal bone cyst

The absence of periosteal reaction and presence of intact cortex make Ewing sarcoma, osteosarcoma or chondrosarcoma unlikely. Fibrous dysplasia is possible but the appearance and location would be atypical. The major differential is a giant cell tumour.

37 Answer D: Ewing sarcoma

Ewing sarcoma is commonest in this age group and in a diaphyseal location. Neuroblastoma microscopically does contain small blue cells but typically locates in the adrenal gland of children. Medulloblastoma is composed of small blue cells but typically is found in posterior fossa of children. Osteoblastoma is essentially a large osteoid osteoma. Chondroblastomas are epiphyseal tumours.

38 Answer A: Medial approach

A medial approach is advocated to avoid the suprapatellar pouch and avoid an intra-articular track. A lateral approach is used for laterally placed masses in lower and upper femur, a posterior approach has greater risk of neurovascular damage and an anterior approach may compromise knee extension. There is no internal approach.

39 Answer D: Prostate

Prostate cancer is well-known for causing osteoblastic metastases. Breast and lung cancer produce mixed lytic and sclerotic metastases. Kidney and thyroid cancers are usually purely lytic.

40 Answer C: Chondroblastoma

The patella is considered an epiphyseal equivalent and hence the same differential applies. Osteosarcomas, osteochondromas and non-ossifying fibromas are metaphyseal lesions. Adamantinomas are diaphyseal.

41 Answer B: Aneurysmal bone cyst

The appearance of fluid-fluid levels on MRI is characteristic and the appearance given on plain film is typical.

42 Answer B: Biopsy, 'extended' curettage and packing with follow-up X-rays

A biopsy is usually performed to confirm the diagnosis and exclude malignancy. Extended curettage is then performed to reduce the risk of recurrence (approx 30%).

43 Answer E: Diaphyseal

44 Answer D: Wide resection and chemotherapy

Wide surgical margins and limb-sparing resection combined with chemotherapy is the most successful regime. Pre- and post-operative chemotherapy significantly improves outcome.

45 Answer A: Chest X-ray

Lung metastases are the most common metastases from sarcomas, including osteogenic sarcomas. He may also need a CT but of the available options a CXR is the best initial test.

46 Answer C: Chondrosarcoma

Chondrosarcoma generally occurs in adults over the age of 60 and the proximal humerus is a common location. 'Popcorn' calcification is a typical radiological sign. Chondroblastoma occurs in a much younger patient population (10–30 years) and typically has a sclerotic border.

47 Answer B: Osteoblastoma

Osteoblastoma, in contrast to many other benign bone lesions, are frequently associated with an extra-cortical mass.

48 Answer E: Osteoid osteoma

This is a typical description of an osteoid osteoma with a central nidus.

49 Answer E: McCune-Albright syndrome

McCune-Albright syndrome is the triad of fibrous dysplasia, café au lait spots and endocrine dysfunction. Bone lesions in fibrous dysplasia typically have a 'ground-glass' appearance. Hand-Schüller-Christian disease is the triad of exophthalmos, diabetes insipidus and lytic skull lesions. In Gardner's syndrome there are multiple neoplasms of bone and intestinal polyps. Letterer-Siwe disease is a severe form of histiocytosis X.

50 Answer A: Fibrous dysplasia

Fibrous dysplasia typically has a ground-glass appearance, a thick sclerotic border and often presents as a result of a pathological fracture.

51 Answer C: Ewing sarcoma

The intermediate signal on T2 is due to the presence of hypercellular tumour combined, which suggests extensive soft-tissue disease, a characteristic feature of Ewing sarcoma. Osteomyelitis can mimic changes of an aggressive bone tumour but is not the most likely diagnosis here. Lymphoma tends to affect older children. Chondroblastoma does occur in this age group but arises in the epiphysis and has a sclerotic rim.

52   Answer E: Giant cell tumour

These are typical findings of a GCT and the age of the patient is also typical. Aneurysmal bone cysts tend to cause more expansion and to be more diaphyseal. Unicameral bone cyst (also known as simple bone cyst), can be mildly expansile but not multiloculated.

53   Answer C: Plasma cells

The patient has multiple myeloma with a high serum globulin.

54   Answer A: Enchondroma

The description is typical. The risk of malignant degeneration in solitary peripheral enchondromas is very small.

55   Answer B: Osteosarcoma

The most common site for osteosarcoma is the distal femur. Pain is worse with activity and with a high ALP the patient is more likely to have lung metastases.

56   Answer C: Giant cell tumour

Giant cell tumours are metaphyseal lesions that extend to the articular surface. They are most common in the third and fourth decades of life. The low signal intensity on T1- and T2-weighted images seen with giant cell tumours is due to haemosiderin deposition. All the other diagnoses have high signal intensity on T2-weighted images.

57   Answer B: Multiple myeloma

Multiple myeloma classically presents with well-demarcated, radiolucent lesions without a sclerotic border which may be symmetrical and may be associated with osteopenia. It would be unusual for prostatic metastases to be so well-defined, lytic and widespread.

58   Answer E: Osteoid osteoma

The appearance of a central nidus with surrounding sclerosis is common. Osteoblastoma tends to have irregular margins and is larger (2–10 cm). Chronic sclerosing osteomyelitis is also usually irregular with more bone destruction and periosteal reaction although it is possible to mistake a sequestrum for the nidus.

59   Answer B: Lymphoma of bone

Of the options listed lymphoma is most likely to have this appearance; in particular it is relatively slow growing. Multiple myeloma is lucent but has no expansion. A sarcoma would also be possible but is not listed.

60   Answer E: Intramedullary

Ependymomas are intramedullary tumours.

61 Answer C: 30–40 years

Haemangiopericytoma is a rare tumour that usually occurs in the soft tissue of the thigh, pelvis or retroperitoneum and presents as a painless slow-growing mass. They may show locally aggressive behaviour.

62 Answer B: Normal surrounding bone, rings and arcs within lesion

63 Answer B: 5–10 years

64 Answer C: Variable signal on T1-weighted images, high signal on T2-weighted images

Haemangiomas return a variable but usually high signal on T1-weighted images and a high signal on T2. They are most commonly found between the ages of 10 and 50.

65 Answer D: L1

Tuberculous spondylitis is also known as Pott disease. It is a destructive process and usually more than one level is affected. It occurs in less than 1% of patients with TB and is due to spread through the paravertebral venous plexus. Other radiological features include: paraspinal infection, demineralisation of endplates, collapse of vertebral body and ivory vertebrae.

66 Answer C: *Staphylococcus aureus*

Brodie's abscesses are more common in children and tend to affect the end of tubular bones, most commonly the distal tibia or femur.

67 Answer C: Holt-Oram syndrome

This is a rare syndrome with autosomal dominant inheritance characterised by radial ray limb anomalies and congenital cardiac disease.

68 Answer D: Chondromalacia patella

This common condition is due to softening of the articular cartilage and is often associated with patella maltracking. It is very often an asymptomatic finding at arthroscopy performed for another reason.

69 Answer D: Supraspinatus

Deltoid is not part of the rotator cuff. Supraspinatus is most frequently injured at or close to its insertion into the humerus.

70 Answer A: None

Enostoses are benign incidental findings that may increase slowly or decrease in size. It could be significant if at a critical load-bearing region but at 7 mm it is unlikely to be clinically relevant in the ilium.

Musculoskeletal and trauma radiology

PAPER 3: ANSWERS AND EXPLANATIONS

1 Answer B: Ankylosing spondylitis (AS)

This is the most likely diagnosis because it affects younger males, with extensive sclerosis and often with erosions. AS can cause both SI joint widening and fusion. Diseases that can cause bilateral symmetrical sacroiliitis include: AS, enteropathic arthropathy, late rheumatoid arthritis, deposition arthropathy and osteitis condensans ilii.

Levine DS, Forbat SM, Saifuddin A. MRI of the axial skeletal manifestations of ankylosing spondylitis. *Clin Radiol.* 2004; **59**(5): 400–13.

2 Answer D: MRI

MRI is 90–100% sensitive and 80% specific for diagnosing symptomatic disease, reflecting death of marrow fat cells. Nuclear medicine scans are 80–85% sensitive, with bone marrow imaging more sensitive than bone imaging. Early disease shows a cold area from interrupted vasculature; late disease shows a 'doughnut' sign, a cold spot with a surrounding ring of increased uptake due to capillary revascularisation, and new bone synthesis. Plain radiographic appearances may be unremarkable in the early stages of AVN. Early diagnosis with MRI is therefore required if the diagnosis is suspected to prevent joint replacement.

3 Answer D: Diminished uptake in medullary RES

Features differ between the acute and healing phase. In medullary infarction, the nutrient artery is involved. In cortical infarction, the nutrient artery and periosteal vessels are affected. In the acute phase of medullary infarction, there are no radiographic changes without cortical involvement and decreased uptake on the bone marrow scan with increased uptake after a collateral circulation is established. In the healing phase (complete healing, fibrosis or calcification) the appearances are of serpiginous or linear calcification peripherally, with dense bone from revascularisation.

4   Answer A: Ossification of patellar ligament

DISH is also known as Forestier disease or ankylosing hyperostosis and is an ossifying diathesis with a proliferation of entheses (bony growths at tendon and ligament insertions). DISH principally affects the spine, pelvis and extremities. The differential diagnosis includes: fluorosis, acromegaly, ankylosing spondylitis and intervertebral osteochondrosis. The features are ossification of patellar ligament, heel spurs, whiskering of the iliac crest and flowing ossification of at least four contiguous vertebral bodies.

5   Answer A: Cartilaginous rest

Cartilaginous rests are round radiolucencies, caused by displaced cartilage in the bone. An enchondroma is a benign cartilaginous lesion. Enchondromatosis, also known as Ollier's disease, is due to derangement of cartilaginous growth, leading to migration of cartilaginous rests from the epiphysis to the metaphysis, where proliferation occurs. It is usually diagnosed in childhood and, in addition to abnormal growth, it is associated with juvenile granulosa cell tumours of the ovary. The main complication is sarcomatous transformation, which is more common in axial rather than appendicular enchondromas. Maffucci's syndrome is similar except that it also involves haemangiomas and lymphangiomas.

6   Answer B: Radionuclide whole body bone scan

Skeletal survey is more appropriate for multiple myeloma screening. Some literature states PSA<20 does not warrant a bone scan although centres vary in their practice. CT of the whole spine is unnecessary, although a targeted study can be useful if there is doubt. Similarly MR can be performed but this should be targeted at areas flagged up by a bone scan. Three-phase bone scans are used for targeted regions to assess for loosening and infection.

7   Answer E: Insufficiency fracture

The 'H' sign is usually diagnostic of a sacral insufficiency fracture. The sacrum can be difficult to assess on conventional radiography and its absence does not exclude pathology.

8   Answer A: Joint space preserved until late in disease

Gout is a disorder of purine metabolism, typically in middle-aged males, with four main parts: hyperuricaemia, deposition of positively birefringent crystals in synovial fluid, deposits of sodium urate in periarticular soft tissues, recurrent episodes of arthritis. It can be primary or secondary. The gouty tophus is pathognomonic histologically. The stages are: asymptomatic hyperuricaemia, acute gouty arthritis, chronic tophaceous gout and gouty nephropathy. Forty-five per cent of affected patients have radiological features, but these features are not seen until 6–12 years after the initial attack. Common locations are: joints, particularly hands and feet, bones, external ear. In the joint, effusion is the earliest sign, with periarticular swelling and preservation of joint space until late in the disease. The attacks are short so there is no periarticular demineralisation. Eccentric erosions are also seen, particularly at the metacarpal bases. Chondrocalcinosis is only seen in 5%.

9 Answer E: Bronchiectasis

Hypertrophic osteoarthropathy is a syndrome of proliferative periostitis of the long bones, digital clubbing and arthralgia. Symptoms include pain and swelling of the wrist and ankles. Non-small-cell lung cancer is the most common malignant association. HOA is cited to be present in 31% of lung cancer patients and often precedes chest symptoms. Ectopic production of growth factors is thought to be the underlying causative factor. Other neoplasia in which HOA is seen include: pulmonary metastases (secondary to breast, nasopharyngeal tumours, renal cell carcinoma, melanoma, osteosarcoma) as well as benign conditions (benign pleural fibroma and bronchiectasis).

10 Answer C: Chondrocalcinosis

Haemochromatosis can be primary (inherited) or secondary (excessive iron absorption in anaemias, myelofibrosis, exogenous administration). Symptoms include: cirrhosis, congestive heart failure, arthritic symptoms. Skeletal features include: generalised osteoporosis, small subchondral cyst-like lesions in the metacarpal heads, arthropathy in 50%, uniform joint space narrowing, enlargement of metacarpal heads, osteophyte formation and chondrocalcinosis in 60%. The differential diagnosis includes: pseudogout, psoriatic arthritis, OA, RA, gout.

11 Answer B: Lead poisoning

The pathology of this involves lead concentrating in the metaphyses of growing bones (distal femur most often, then ends of tibia and then distal radius). These are known as lead lines, occur in a chronic state of poisoning and are growth arrests. The differential diagnosis is healed rickets, leukaemia, scurvy and normal increased density in infants less than three years of age. As lead and calcium are used interchangeably by bone, lead deposition occurs in high concentrations in growing bones, with the greatest concentration in the metaphyses, particularly those in the distal femora, ends of the tibiae and distal radii, as these are the parts of the skeleton that grow most rapidly. Risk factors include: exposure to lead paint, especially in old houses, eye makeup, occupational exposure.

12 Answer E: Fibrosis of overlying skin is typical

Melorheostosis is a nonhereditary disease of unknown aetiology, which has a slow course in adults and a rapid course in children. It has multiple associations: osteopoikilosis, osteopathia striata, blood vessel malformations. It is generally present in one limb or in a dermatomal distribution. Physical signs include thickening and fibrosis of the overlying skin and typical features include the 'dripping candle wax' sign – blotches of sclerosis along a tubular bone, from proximal to distal. It can cross joints leading to flexion contractures or fusion. In addition, genu varus, genu valgus and limb length discrepancy can occur.

Bansal A. The dripping candle wax sign. *Radiology*. 2008; **246**(2): 638–40.

13 Answer B: Loose bodies

The patient usually experiences a warm, painless joint, usually with a joint effusion, narrowed joint space, calcification in the soft tissues, and fragmentation of subchondral bone. Juxta-articular osteoporosis is not usually seen unless the joint is infected. Dense subchondral bone (sclerosis), Degeneration, Destruction of articular cortex, Deformity ('pencil points' of metatarsal heads), Debris and Dislocation is one way of helping remember the findings.

14 Answer B: Still disease

This is essentially rheumatoid arthritis in patients younger than 16 and is more common in females. Still disease is systemic and may be polyarticular or pauci-articular. Typical findings include 'balloon epiphyses', 'gracile bones', rectangular phalanges and ribbon ribs. Large joints tend to be involved first. Other differences from rheumatoid arthritis are a late onset of bony changes, more ankylosis and widening of the metaphyses.

15 Answer B: Fibrous dysplasia

There are at least 10 causes but the four most common are: osteomalacia, fibrous dysplasia, osteogenesis imperfecta, Paget's. Pseudofractures are the same as Looser lines or osteoid seams, and are insufficiency fractures and non-union. They occur at sites of mechanical stress such as where vessels enter bone. They tend to be bilateral and symmetric at right angles to the bone margin. The pathognomonic sign is a 2–3 mm stripe of lucency at right angles to the cortex (osteoid seam).

16 Answer B: Transient osteoporosis

This is a self-limiting disease of unknown aetiology. A characteristic is loss of subchondral cortex of the femoral head and neck region. Unlike other forms of arthritis, there is no joint space narrowing or subchondral bone collapse. Radiographic features include a joint effusion, increased uptake on bone scans, diffuse marrow oedema of the femoral head and neck (MR) and pathological fractures. There is usually spontaneous recovery within two to six months, but recurrence elsewhere is possible.

17 Answer E: Posteromedial

In the preslip stages there is widening of the growth plate with irregularity. Posteromedial displacement occurs in an acute slip when the epiphysis may appear smaller due to posterior displacement. The slip is usually best seen on the lateral view.

18 Answer B: Tuberous sclerosis

Tuberous sclerosis is an autosomal-dominant condition that presents with seizures, mental retardation and skin lesions. There are multisystem features: CNS, renal, skeletal, pulmonary and cardiac. Skeletal lesions are present in up to half of patients.

19 Answer C: Bony union across middle facet

Tarsal coalition is an abnormal fibrous, cartilaginous or osseous fusion of two or more tarsal bones. It affects 1–2% of the population and is thought to be present at birth with a fibrous band, which later ossifies leading to diagnosis in late teens/early adulthood. It is generally an incidental finding, but can be associated with hindfoot pain. MR can distinguish between cartilaginous and bony unions.

20 Answer B: Ochronosis

Ochronosis or alkaptonuria is due to an inherited enzyme defect (homogentisic acid oxidase) and results in deposition of black pigment in cartilage. The features described are typical and affected individuals may also suffer from renal and cardiac failure.

21 Answer D: Radiotherapy

Processes that appear high signal on T2 include: osteoporotic vertebral collapse, radiotherapy, haemangiomas, type 1 and 2 vertebral end plate changes. Both lytic and sclerotic metastases return low signal on T1, with lytic metastases returning high signal on T2 and sclerotic low signal on T2. Myeloma can appear low signal after treatment. Lymphoma and Gaucher's disease tend to be isointense on T2-weighted imaging.

22 Answer C: Contrast-enhanced CT

Multidetector CT imaging is the gold standard for diagnosing and assessing the extent of renal injury, peri-renal haemorrhage, extravasation of urine, pedicle injury, and associated solid-organ injury. Indications include blunt trauma with (macroscopic or microscopic) haematuria and hypotension, polytrauma, rapid deceleration and penetrating injury.

Bent C. Urological injuries following trauma. *Clin Radiol* 2008; **63**(12): 1361–71.

23 Answer E: Retrograde urethrography

Retrograde urethrography is still widely advocated for excluding urethral trauma. Advanced trauma and life-support guidelines consider any of the following as indicators of possible urethral injury: 1 blood at the urethral meatus; 2 perineal ecchymoses; 3 blood in the scrotum; 4 inability to void; 5 elevation of the prostate on digital rectal examination; 6 pelvic fracture.

24 Answer D: MRI within 24 hours

There is still some controversy over whether MRI or scintigraphy are the most sensitive modalities for scaphoid fracture detection, but most authorities would accept that imaging within 24 hours is optimal and scintigraphy is most sensitive at 4–5 days post-injury.

Beeres JP. Early magnetic resonance imaging compared with bone scintigraphy in suspected scaphoid fractures. *J Bone Joint Surg Br*. 2008; **90**(9): 1205–9.

25 Answer B: CT head

There is no scope for a skull X-ray in head trauma. An urgent CT head is mandatory and can delineate fractures and acute haemorrhage very well.

National Institute for Clinical Excellence. *Investigation for Clinically Important Brain Injury: NICE guideline 56*. London: NIHCE; 2007. www.nice.org/guidance/CG056

Selection of adults for CT scan: urgent scan if any of the following (results within 1 hour)

- GCS<13 when first assessed or GCS<15 two hours after injury
- Suspected open or depressed skull fracture
- Signs of base of skull fracture
- Post-traumatic seizure
- Focal neurological deficit
- >1 episode of vomiting
- Coagulopathy + any amnesia or LOC since injury

A CT scan is also recommended (within eight hours of injury) if there is either more than 30 minutes of amnesia of events before impact or any amnesia or LOC since injury if one of the following applies: Aged ≥65 years, coagulopathy or on warfarin or a dangerous mechanism of injury (i.e. RTA as pedestrian, RTA – ejected from car, fall >1 m or >5 stairs).

Selection of children (under 16 years) for CT scan: urgent scan if any of the following:

- witnessed loss of consciousness >5 minutes
- amnesia (antegrade or retrograde) >5 minutes
- Abnormal drowsiness
- ≥3 Discrete episodes of vomiting
- clinical suspicion of NAI
- post-traumatic seizure (no PMH epilepsy)
- GCS <14 in emergency room
- (paediatric GCS<15 if aged <1)
- suspected open or depressed skull fracture or tense fontanelle
- signs of base of skull fracture
- focal neurological deficit
- aged <1 – bruise, swelling or laceration on head >5 cm
- dangerous mechanism of injury (high speed RTA, fall from >3 m, high speed projectile).

26 Answer D: Visible posterior fat pad

Elevation of the anterior fat pad is abnormal, but it is often visible without elevation as it sits in the shallow coronoid fossa of the humerus. Visualisation of the posterior fat pad is almost always abnormal, as it normally lies hidden within the deeper olecranon fossa.

27 Answer E: Fracture of surgical neck of humerus

The most likely injury in this context of falling on an outstretched arm, particularly in a patient with an osteoporotic humerus, is a fracture of the surgical neck, which is the point of weakness and is most easily fractured by an axial force. A fracture of the deltoid tuberosity is rare and would usually only occur with an avulsion by the deltoid tendon. The anatomical neck is not commonly fractured. Posterior dislocations are not common, occurring classically in the context of an epileptic fit or electrocution.

28 Answer B: Fracture of left seventh rib posteriorly

Injuries suggestive of NAI include: metaphyseal corner, posterior rib, scapula and spinous process fractures, subependymal haemorrhages, bruises of different ages, and fractures not consistent with the expected stage of development of the child. For this reason, spiral fractures of the long bones would be consistent with an injury sustained by a walking toddler, but would be unusual below 18 months of age. Greenstick fractures are common in all children and are not in themselves suspicious for NAI. A supracondylar fracture is plausible if the history is suggestive; for example, falling from a climbing frame. Posterior rib fractures and metaphyseal corner fractures are particular common fractures in the setting of NAI.

29 Answer B: Triangular fibrocartilage

Injuries to the TFC are a frequent cause of ulnar-sided wrist pain. The ulnar side of the wrist is supported by the TFC, which articulates with the lunate and triquetral distally. Tears are most commonly associated with a positive ulnar variance but may occur as a result of direct trauma; for example forced ulnar deviation on hitting a ball with a cricket bat. The extensor carpi ulnaris tendon sheath, dorsal and volar radioulnar ligaments and ulnocarpal ligaments are all part of the TFC complex. However, it is the TFC proper (articular disc) that is the most commonly injured structure in the complex.

30 Answer E: Osteochondritis dissecans

Osteochondritis dissecans typically affects the lateral surface of the medial femoral condyle in adolescent males but may also involve the weight-bearing surface of the lateral femoral condyle, tibia or patella. A fragment may separate from the underlying bone and present as an intra-articular loose body (approximately 50% of cases) with pain, swelling and locking of the knee. The condition is bilateral in 20–25% of cases. Osgood-Schlatter disease is the eponym for traction apophysitis of the tibial tuberosity. Subchondral sclerosis and cysts are hallmarks of degenerative arthritis, although the patient's age makes this much less likely.

31 Answer D: Torus fracture of distal third of the radius

Common fractures in immature skeletons are torus (buckle) and greenstick fractures which occur due to the softer nature of immature bone, which is more likely to buckle on itself than fracture completely with moderate force. With greater force, a greenstick fracture can occur in which one cortex is fractured while the other bends. In both cases an excellent recovery is possible with closed reduction for six weeks. Monteggia fracture-dislocation is a fracture of the proximal ulna in conjunction with a dislocation of the distal radio-ulnar joint. It is rare, seen with significant trauma and not typical in a child. Salter-Harris type III fractures are also rare. The more common type of Salter-Harris fracture is a type II fracture. Comminuted distal fractures are not usually seen in children and would require a significant force to occur.

32 Answer C: There is a sensitivity of 40% for the detection of solid-organ injuries

The focused abdominal sonography for trauma (FAST) evaluation is usually performed on patients with blunt abdominal trauma to look for free fluid in the abdomen and pelvis. This usually includes sonography of the right upper quadrant, including the hepatorenal fossa; the left upper quadrant, including the perisplenic region; the right and left paracolic gutters; and the pelvis. Free fluid will gravitate to the most dependent portion of the pelvis and therefore may be missed if the patient has an empty bladder. In some instances an examination of the epigastrium is also performed. Other components of the examination include an intercostal or subdiaphragmatic view of the heart. Examination of the chest is performed if there has been chest as well as abdominal trauma. A few studies cite some benefit from serial measurements of ascitic fluid.

McGahan JP, Richards J, Gillen M. The focused abdominal sonography for trauma scan: pearls and pitfalls. *J Ultrasound Med.* 2002; **21**(7): 789–800.

33 Answer D: L1

A 'Chance' fracture describes a horizontal fracture through the spinous process, laminae, pedicles and vertebral body from a hyperflexion-distraction type of injury. It classically occurs as a result of deceleration affecting rear-seat passengers restrained in lap seatbelts and the thoraco-lumbar junction is the most common site of injury. A CT scan is the best modality for evaluating these fractures and other associated injuries (50% incidence of abdominal injuries with Chance fracture). Immobilisation is generally adequate treatment for these fractures; however, kyphosis of greater than 20 degrees is an indication for surgical fixation and spinal cord decompression as there may be instability.

34 Answer E: Medial meniscus, anterior cruciate ligament tear and Segond fracture

A Segond fracture is a capsular avulsion fracture seen at the lateral aspect of the proximal tibia and is often associated with high-energy sporting and ski injuries. There is usually associated ACL and meniscal injury and a medial tibial plateau impaction fracture may be present. A reverse Segond fracture is an avulsion fracture of the medial tibial margin. It is strongly associated with medial meniscal and PCL tears and caused by severe hyperextension and valgus stress.

35 Answer E: Axillary nerve

Axillary nerve function is assessed pre- and post-shoulder relocation by testing for sensation in the 'regimental patch' area of skin in the upper arm and deltoid power (shoulder abduction). The nerve is at risk of damage from a dislocated humeral head where it lies close to the inferior joint capsule.

36 Answer E: Prostate carcinoma

Elevated alkaline phosphatase in elderly men must raise the suspicion of bony metastases from prostate carcinoma, which is the commonest cause of sclerotic metastases.

37 Answer B: Chondrosarcoma

Both chondrosarcoma and osteosarcoma commonly present with paraneoplastic hyperglycaemia (85% of cases with central chondrosarcoma, 25% of osteosarcoma) but the patient's age and the site are more typical for a chondrosarcoma.

38 Answer D: Giant cell tumour

Giant cell tumours are almost invariably epiphyseal although they may extend to involve the metaphysis. They occur almost exclusively in those with closed epiphyses and are eccentric with a non-sclerotic margin.

39 Answer A: Osteitis fibrosa cystica

Osteitis fibrosa cystica is caused by an excess of PTH causing increased osteoclastic resorption of bone. It is seen in people with hyperparathyroidism and can present with headaches and bone pain. Fibrous dysplasia, osteochondroma, Paget's disease of bone and giant cell tumour are not associated with disorders of calcium metabolism.

40 Answer B: Well-defined lucent lesion with sclerotic rim in the metaphysis

Chondromyxoid fibromas generally occur between the ages of 10 and 30 years. Internal calcification is uncommon.

41 Answer D: Giant cell tumour (GCT)

GCTs are characteristically well defined with a non-sclerotic margin and are most frequently seen in young adults aged between 20 and 40 years. Most GCTs occur in the long bones, but a number do occur in the spine where they tend to affect younger patients and to be three to four times more common in the sacrum than rest of spine.

42 Answer A: Epiphyseal

Giant cell tumours are usually epiphyseal in a sub-articular location but may extend from the epiphysis to involve the metaphysis. Ninety-seven per cent occur after closure of the epiphyses.

43 Answer E: Osteosarcoma

Osteosarcoma may rarely arise in Paget's disease through malignant degeneration. Sclerotic metastases are probably more common even in someone known to have Paget's but are usually multifocal and would rarely involve only one part of one bone.

44 Answer E: 10–20%

Osteosarcoma has a very poor prognosis once metastases are present.

45 Answer C: Osteoid osteoma

Osteoid osteoma is a benign bone tumour composed of osteoid and woven bone that usually affects young individuals. They are small tumours (less than 2 cm in diameter) with a central nidus in which prostaglandin E2 is elevated. This has been suggested to be the cause of the pain experienced and explains the typical history of relief with salicylates.

46 Answer A: Location in the posterior elements

An osteoblastoma is histologically identical to an osteoid osteoma but usually larger and the classical description is of a well-defined expansile lesion in the posterior elements of the spine. Around 80% of cases present before 30 years of age and a sclerotic rim is usually present. There is, however, a wide variety of possible appearances including cortical thinning and a soft-tissue mass which can resemble a malignant process.

47 Answer E: Osteoid osteoma

The femoral neck is the most common location for osteoid osteomas.

48 Answer B: Giant cell tumour

Giant cell tumours are typically epiphyseal and the 'soap bubble' appearance is characteristic. More destruction would be expected with the other options.

49 Answer D: Osteoid osteoma

Osteoid osteoma has a typical double-density sign of a nidus with surrounding activity due to the reactive sclerosis. With a stress fracture of the femoral neck it is unusual to see the double-density sign. Brodie's abscess usually has a more uniform pattern of radiotracer uptake. A simple bone cyst has no uptake on a bone scan.

50 Answer A: Mazabraud's syndrome

Mazabraud's syndrome is the rare association of fibrous dysplasia with intramuscular myxoma and is an important differential for a soft-tissue mass with lytic bone lesions.

51   Answer B: Chondrosarcoma

Chondrosarcoma tends to occur in those over 40 and the median age at presentation is 45 years. Giant cell tumour has a peak incidence in the third and fourth decades, and has a female preponderance. Osteosarcoma is most often seen in the first to third decades of life, although there is a second peak after the age of 60 due to Paget's disease. Aneurysmal bone cyst is most commonly present in the second and third decades and osteoid osteoma in the first three decades.

52   Answer A: Femur

The most common location is the femur followed by the ilium, tibia, humerus, fibula sacrum and ribs in that order.

53   Answer D: Metaphyseal and diaphyseal

Approximately two-thirds of Ewing sarcomas affect long bones and half of these are centred in the metadiaphysis.

54   Answer D: Osteogenic sarcoma

Osteogenic sarcoma is the most common primary malignant bone tumour. It classically affects adolescents with a second peak in incidence after the age of 60 due to Paget's disease. The typical presentation is with pain of several weeks' duration, commonly with activity. The most common bones involved are the femur and tibia with the majority of lesions occurring around the knee. An important differential is osteomyelitis.

55   Answer D: Simple bone cyst

56   Answer D: Chondroblastoma

Chondroblastomas are usually spherical, well-defined lesions in an epiphyseal location and with a fine sclerotic margin. Florid marrow oedema surrounding the lesion is also a typical feature. Aneurysmal bone cysts have a low signal rim on both T1- and T2-weighted MRI images but bone marrow oedema is not typical. Giant cell tumours are rare in children and their margins are not sclerotic. Chondrosarcomas are epiphyseal but rare in this age group.

57   Answer C: Metaphysis

Enchondromas are metaphyseal, although they may affect the epiphysis after closure of the growth plate.

58   Answer C: Alpha feta protein

Sacrococcygeal teratoma is the most common solid tumour occurring in the newborn and alpha feta protein is raised in malignant teratomas. It is more common in girls and is associated with other congenital anomalies such as spinal dysraphism, sacral agenesis, hydronephrosis, imperforate anus and gastroschisis. Sacrococcygeal teratomas are typically mixed cystic/solid and on MRI they are heterogeneous with high signal on T1-weighted images. The older the child is at presentation the more likely the tumour is to be malignant.

59 Answer A: Expansile, lytic lesion

Thyroid and renal cell carcinoma metastases are nearly always osteolytic. Other causes of lytic metastases include melanoma, lung and breast carcinomas. The most common causes of sclerotic metastases are prostatic, breast, colonic and bladder carcinomas in addition to melanoma and soft-tissue sarcomas.

60 Answer C: Thoracic spine

Almost two-thirds occur in the thoracic spinal cord, although half involve the cervical cord as they usually extend over a long region of cord (approximately seven segments on average).

61 Answer B: Anterior cruciate ligament tear

The PCL is bowed due to posterior translation of the femur on the tibia. There is very often an associated meniscal tear.

62 Answer C: Metacarpals

The majority occur in the small tubular bones of the hand.

63 Answer B: 10–30 years

Three-quarters will be within this range.

64 Answer C: Hepatoma

The patient has haemochromatosis and cirrhosis is common. Cardiac failure is also a common cause of death. Females present later if at all due to the protective effect of menstruation.

65 Answer D: Triple phase Tc-99m methylene-diphosphonate (MDP) bone scan

Plain radiography is often used initially but generally only shows changes late on in the process, including endosteal and periosteal reaction. Triple-phase bone scintigraphy detects osteoblastic activity, which occurs during remodelling and is very sensitive. False positive results can occur in infection, osteonecrosis and neoplasia. CT is less sensitive than bone scintigraphy and MRI but it is useful in areas where plain film is limited and is more sensitive than plain film or MRI for detecting cortical fractures.

Datir AP, Saini A, Connell D, *et al.* Stress-related bone injuries with emphasis on MRI. *Clin Radiol.* 2007; **62**(9): 828–36.

66 Answer D: Knee

Eighty per cent of cases occur in the knee and are usually monoarticular.

67 Answer C: Bankart lesion

This is a tear of the anterior glenoid labrum and may be associated with a Hill Sachs defect in the posterolateral surface of the humeral head.

68 Answer D: Patella

This rare syndrome is due to in utero exposure to a toxin such as thalidomide. It is often associated with fibular hemimelia and absence of the patella.

69 Answer D: Autosomal recessive

He had progeria, which often presents with absence of the adolescent growth spurt and beginning of premature ageing.

70 Answer D: Rectus femoris

Gastrointestinal and hepatobiliary radiology

PAPER 1: ANSWERS AND EXPLANATIONS

1   Answer A: Breast

The most common direct extension to the oesophagus is from the bronchus. The most common metastases from a distant primary are from breast, which are usually submucosal.

2   Answer D: Plummer-Vinson syndrome

Plummer-Vinson syndrome is characterised by oesophageal webs, iron deficiency anaemia, stomatitis, glossitis, dysphagia, thyroid disorders and spoon-shaped nails. An oesophageal web is usually seen near the cricopharyngeus and arises at right angles from the anterior oesophageal wall. It is usually asymptomatic unless there is severe stenosis.

3   Answer B: Serious liver disease

Peritonitis, post-operative ileus and acute pancreatitis are relative contraindications.

4   Answer C: Epiploic appendagitis

Epiploic appendagitis (EA) is uncommon and is due to inflammation of one of the 100 or so epiploic/omental appendages that arise from the serosal surface of the colon. Histology shows acute infarction with fat necrosis, inflammation and thrombosed vessels with haemorrhagic suffusion, but if recognised on CT it can usually be treated conservatively with spontaneous resolution within two weeks. CT appearances resolve by six months. The typical patient is a male in their forties.

5   Answer C: Herpes oesophagitis

6   Answer C: Diffuse oesophageal spasm

The classic presentation of diffuse oesophageal spasm is with severe intermittent pain while swallowing. These swallow appearances are characteristic and extremely high pressures are seen on manometry.

7   Answer C: Squamous cell carcinoma

Squamous cell carcinoma in 95%, associated with head and neck carcinoma, smoking, alcohol, achalasia and Lye ingestion. Adenocarcinoma (5%) usually occurs in the lower oesophagus at the GOJ and is associated with Barrett's oesophagus. It is increasing in frequency.

8   Answer B: Aberrant right subclavian artery

The right subclavian artery normally arises from the brachiocephalic trunk bifurcation. An aberrant right subclavian is the last branch of the aortic arch distal to the left subclavian and indents the oesophagus posteriorly.

9   Answer C: Oesophageal intramural pseudodiverticulosis

The characteristic features of oesophageal intramural pseudodiverticulosis on barium swallow include multiple tiny 'floating' barium collections and oesophageal structuring. In 90% of cases it is associated with diabetes, alcoholism, oesophagitis and structuring.

10   Answer C: Primary achalasia

Primary achalasia is characterised by failure of organised peristalsis and relaxation of the lower oesophageal sphincter. Imaging features include: megaoesophagus, absent primary peristalsis, nonperistaltic contractions and 'rat-tail'/'bird-beak' oesophagus.

11   Answer E: Pneumomediastinum

Spontaneous oesophageal perforation (Boerhaave's syndrome) typically results from persistent vomiting following an alcoholic binge. Radiographic features typically include: pneumomediastinum, pleural effusion and mediastinal haematoma.

12   Answer C: Meckel's diverticulum

Meckel's diverticulum is due to persistence of the omphalomesenteric duct, which normally obliterates in utero. Fifty per cent contain ectopic mucosa, which is usually gastric but may be pancreatic or colonic. This can demonstrate technetium uptake similar to normal stomach mucosa. It is therefore very important that the entire abdomen is imaged on the camera simultaneously to demonstrate simultaneous uptake.

13   Answer B: T4a N3 M0

14   Answer D: Pyloric transverse diameter 15 mm and presence of the cervix sign

The 'cervix sign' is the indentation of muscle mass on the fluid-filled antrum in longitudinal section and is seen in pyloric stenosis. Maximal dimensions of the canal on USS are 17 mm in length, 3 mm wall thickness, 13 mm in diameter and volume of 1.4 cu cm.

15   Answer D: Limited to the serosa

16 Answer C: Atrophic gastritis

The incidence of atrophic gastritis increases with age and symptoms may include epigastric pain and early satiety. Radiological features are a narrow tubular stomach and a reduction in the normal gastric folds.

17 Answer C: Clotted blood

Serum: 0–20 HU, Fresh unclotted blood: 30–45 HU, Clotted blood: 60–100 HU: Active arterial extravasation >180 HU (on enhanced scan).

18 Answer A: Crohn's disease

Although Crohn's disease more frequently affects the small bowel, involvement of the stomach and duodenum occurs in up to 10% of patients. Typical appearances include aphthoid ulcers, erosions, cobblestone mucosa and thickened duodenal folds.

19 Answer D: Scirrhous cancer

The listed radiological features are typical of linitis plastica (leather bottle stomach) of which scirrhous cancer is the most common cause. Other causes include: other tumours (lymphoma, metastases, pancreatic carcinoma), inflammation (erosive gastritis, radiation therapy), infiltrative disease (sarcoid, amyloid, intramural haematoma) and infection (TB, syphilis).

20 Answer A: Adhesions

21 Answer B: Liver

Duodenal injury is frequently associated with injury to other abdominal structures. The pattern of these associated injuries varies between blunt and penetrating trauma:

blunt trauma: pancreas > liver > spleen > colon > small bowel > kidney.
penetrating trauma: liver > pancreas > small bowel > kidney > colon > spleen.

22 Answer A: Jejunal injury with disruption of the bowel wall

The most common site of traumatic small bowel injury is the anti-mesenteric border of the proximal jejunum. Blunt abdominal trauma causing hollow viscous injuries occurred in conjunction with multiple trauma in approximately 70% of cases. Bubbles of gas are often seen close to the affected segment; wall disruption will most likely be present if free gas is present.

23 Answer A: Ileocolic intussusception

This is a classic age and history for intussusceptions and the most common site type is ileocolic.

24 Answer A: Sand-like nodules (approximately 1 mm) in non-dilated small bowel

Whipple disease characteristically causes sand-like nodules in a non-dilated small bowel.

25 Answer B: Normal study

26 Answer E: Ulcers with elevated margins following lymphoid follicles

Gastrointestinal tuberculosis most commonly affects the ileocaecal region and may mimic Crohn's disease. Large shallow, linear, stellate ulcers with margins following the orientation of lymphoid follicles are characteristic.

27 Answer A: Reversal of jejunal and ileal fold patterns

28 Answer C: Transverse colon

The transverse colon is the area of bowel where these changes are most commonly seen, probably because it is the least dependent part in the supine position. A mean dilatation of 80 mm is seen in florid cases, but anything over 55 mm is worrying. Sometimes ulceration is so extensive that no mucosal islands remain.

29 Answer D: Intersphincteric

An intersphincteric fistula passes through the internal sphincter and then between the internal and external to the perianal area.

30 Answer E: Bowel distension to the splenic flexure

Bowel distension of the splenic flexure (i.e. the perfusion territory of the superior mesenteric artery) is seen in approximately 40–45% of cases. The other options are all features of ischaemia but are not specific to the superior mesenteric artery territory.

31 Answer C: Turcot syndrome

Turcot syndrome is an autosomal recessive disease characterised by colonic polyposis and central nervous system tumours especially supratentorial glioblastoma and occasionally medulloblastomas. Malignant transformation of the polyps is expected.

32 Answer B: T2, N2, M0.

33 Answer B: MRI pelvis and CT chest

34 Answer D: MRI pelvis

MRI is now the modality of choice for recurrent perianal sepsis as it can delineate the anatomy and identify collections and fistulae.

35 Answer E: *Shigella*

The pattern of colonic involvement can give useful clues to the causative organism in infectious colitis. Organisms that cause colitis limited to the right colon include *Shigella* and *Salmonella*.

36 Answer B: Ascites

CT is abnormal in 60% of cases of pseudomembranous colitis. Marked colonic wall thickening is the commonest manifestation. Ascites occurs in 35%.

37 Answer E: Decrease in hepatic T2 signal on MR

Haemochromatosis can be primary or secondary. The primary form shows autosomal recessive inheritance and usually presents after middle age, particularly in women where menstruation is protective. Hepatomegaly and hyperpigmentation are seen in 90%. Diabetes can occur in up to 30% secondary to pancreatic beta cell damage. Significant signal loss on T2WI is very characteristic.

38 Answer B: Grade II laceration

39 Answer C: *Echinococcus*

40 Answer B: Haemangioma

Hepatic haemangioma are the commonest benign liver tumours. They are typically hyperechoic on ultrasound and demonstrate centripetal enhancement with delayed 'fill-in' on contrast-enhanced CT. Enhancing focal liver lesions can be usefully characterised according to the phase of their enhancement. Other lesions that show delayed (equilibrium phase) enhancement include: cholangiocarcinoma, solitary fibrous tumour and treated metastases.

41 Answer E: Uptake of hepatobiliary contrast

Reticuloendothelial contrast agents, such as Ferrixan, carboxydextran-coated iron oxide nanoparticles (Resovist®) are taken up by both focal nodular hyperplasia (FNH) and adenoma. Hepatobiliary contrast agents, such as Gadolinium-Benzyloxypropionic tetra-acetate (Gd-BOPTA or MultiHance®) are not taken up by adenoma.

42 Answer C: Haemochromatosis

Causes of increased liver attenuation pre-intravenous contrast include: haemochromatosis, haemosiderosis, iron overload, glycogen storage disease and amiodarone treatment.

43 Answer D: Schistosomiasis

The described ultrasound appearances are typical of schistosomiasis. Radiological features rarely develop until the late stages and are signs of cirrhosis and fibrosis. Patients are at a significantly increases risk of hepatocellular carcinoma (HCC).

44 Answer C: Echogenic material in the portal vein lumen

Echogenic material in the portal vein lumen (67%), increased in portal vein diameter (57%), portosystemic collateral circulation (48%), enlargement of a thrombosed portal vein above 15 mm (38%).

45 Answer E: Malignant melanoma

Malignant melanoma is the most common primary that metastases to the spleen. Malignant melanoma is more common in fair skinned individuals and those that spend a significant amount of time outdoors.

46 Answer B: Liver > spleen > muscle

Signal intensity is related to ratio of red to white pulp. Under eight months of age spleen < liver on T1 and T2 due to red pulp. In children and adults on T1 liver > spleen > muscle, and on T2 spleen > liver.

47 Answer D: Nuclear medicine studies

Splenosis is autotransplantation of splenic fragments post trauma and is best seen with 99 mRBC or 99 mTc sulphur colloid studies.

48 Answer B: Fungal

Microabscesses account for 26% of splenic abscesses. Immunocompromised patients are predisposed to fungal infection particularly due to *Candida*, *Aspergillus* and *Cryptococcus*.

49 Answer B: Haematogenous spread

Splenic abscesses are uncommon and are more prevalent in patients with sickle cell disease, diabetes and the immunocompromised. The causative organism is frequently fungal and includes: *Candida*, *Aspergillus* and *Cryptococcus*. Seventy-five per cent occur due to haematogenous spread of infection; the remaining 25% occur secondary to splenic infarction or penetrating trauma.

50 Answer A: Beneath the left lobe of liver

Most frequent locations in descending order are beneath left lobe of liver, intra-hepatic, retrohepatic, within the falciform ligament, within the interlobar fissure, suprahepatic, and within the anterior abdominal wall.

51 Answer C: Cholesterol

Seventy per cent of gallstones are either made up completely or partly of cholesterol. Thirty per cent are black pigment stones made up of predominantly calcium bilirubinate.

52 Answer B: 15%

Porcelain gallbladder is rare but is associated with chronic cholecystitis. The incidence of carcinoma has been reported at 10–30%, therefore cholecystectomy is often advised.

53 Answer D: Acute cholecystitis

54 Answer D: Injury to the duct of Luschka

An accessory biliary duct can be injured despite good visualisation of the CBD.

55 Answer C: Shrunken gallbladder mimicking a pseudodiverticulum of duodenal bulb.

Ninety per cent of cholecystoduodenal fistulae are associated with perforation due to gallstones. Radiological appearances include pneumobilia and the presence of a shrunken gallbladder mimicking a diverticulum of the duodenal bulb.

56 Answer B: Caroli's disease

Caroli's disease is a rare congenital condition with multifocal segmental cystic dilatation of the large intrahepatic bile ducts, which communicates with the biliary tree.

57 Answer B: Klatskin tumour

Hilar cholangiocarcinoma (Klatskin tumour) is a common cause of biliary obstruction in older patients. Lack of communication between the left and right-sided intrahepatic ducts and normal-calibre extrahepatic ducts are typical findings. Apart from the ductal abnormalities CT findings may be subtle. The tumour mass is often isodense and may show delayed enhancement.

58 Answer C: Primary biliary cirrhosis

This is a chronic non-supperative cholangitis and is associated with autoimmune disorders including rheumatoid arthritis, scleroderma, and Hashimoto's thyroiditis. Sixty-six to one hundred per cent have Sjögren's syndrome symptoms. CT signs include dilated intrahepatic ducts that do not appear to communicate with the main ducts and a hyperattenuating hypertrophied caudate lobe (in 98%) surrounded by hypoattenuating rind-like right lobe (pseudotumour) with a shrunken lateral left lobe.

59 Answer B: Endoscopic ultrasound

Eighty-five per cent staging accuracy.

60 Answer D: MRI liver

Although these may be simple cysts, they should not cause left lobar atrophy or right lobar intrahepatic duct dilatation. There must be a concern of an isodense malignancy at the porta and MRI should be the next investigation.

61 Answer D: Congenital biliary atresia

It is best diagnosed with cholescintigraphy which shows good hepatic uptake but no biliary excretion. Triangular fibrous cord at porta hepatis seen on ultrasound is pathognomonic.

62 Answer D: Pancreatic abscess

Pancreatic abscesses usually occur two to four weeks after onset of severe acute pancreatitis. It is seen as a fluid collection close to the pancreas itself, the most common organism is *E. coli* and 30–50% contain gas. Patients are usually generally unwell and have symptoms and signs of sepsis with raised inflammatory markers. Pseudocysts take over four weeks to develop and rarely contain gas.

63 Answer E: Serous cystadenoma of the pancreas

A serous cystadenoma of the pancreas is a benign lobulated neoplasm composed of innumerable small cysts 1–20 mm. The mass is usually lobulated with a mean size of 5 cm. Any part of the pancreas can be affected but it has slight predominance for the head and neck. The pancreatic duct can be displaced, encased or obstructed. A prominent central stellate scar is characteristic and there is a known association with Von Hippel-Lindau syndrome.

64 Answer A: Annular pancreas

Annular pancreas is a relatively common congenital anomaly wherein a ring of normal pancreatic tissue encircles the duodenum secondary to the abnormal migration of the ventral pancreas. It is associated with other congenital abnormalities in 75%; including Down syndrome. In a neonate it usually presents with duodenal obstruction and the obstruction is at D2 in 85% of cases.

65 Answer E: Demonstrating intraductal stones not surrounded by fluid

Visualising intraductal stones not surrounded by fluid can be difficult with MRI as there is no fluid contrast to outline the filling defect.

Miller FH, Keppke AL, Wadhwa A, *et al*. MRI of pancreatitis and its complications: part 2, chronic pancreatitis. *Am J Roentgenol*. 2004; **183**(6): 1645–52.

66 Answer A: Acute rejection

These are classic features of acute rejection. Clinically, the patient may have focal tenderness over the transplant.

67 Answer E: Junction of body and tail

68 Answer E: Diffuse pancreatic atrophy

69 Answer B: Gastrinoma

Gastrinoma associated with peptic ulceration (Zollinger-Ellison syndrome) is the second most common functioning islet cell tumour. VIPoma is rare and not associated with peptic ulceration. Other functioning islet cell tumours include: insulinoma (commonest functional tumour), somatostatinoma and glucagonoma.

70 Answer E: Radiation enteritis

Radiological changes appear up to one to two years after radiation. The ileum is the most common part of the bowel affected. There is often increased attenuation of the mesentery.

Gastrointestinal and hepatobiliary radiology

PAPER 2: ANSWERS AND EXPLANATIONS

1 Answer B: Endoscopic ultrasound

Endoscopic ultrasound can identify the five separate layers of the oesophageal wall.

2 Answer D: Oesophageal varices

3 Answer A: Rigid endoscope rectal biopsy three days ago

Absolute contraindications to double-contrast barium enema include: toxic megacolon, pseudomembranous colitis and rectal biopsy (within previous five days via rigid endoscope or within previous 24 hours via flexible endoscope). Relative contraindications include: incomplete bowel preparation, recent barium meal and patient frailty.

4 Answer C: Phaeochromocytoma

Contraindications to glucagon administration include: phaeochromocytoma, insulinoma and glucagonoma. Myasthenia gravis, prostatic enlargement and pyloric stenosis are contraindications to Buscopan® administration.

5 Answer E: 'Yo-Yo' motion of the barium

Tertiary oesophageal contractions are non-propulsive motor events characterised by disordered up and down movement of the bolus without clearing of the oesophagus.

6 Answer B: Fixed transverse folds with stepladder appearance of distal oesophagus

The fixed folds are due to the scarring and are often in a transverse orientation. Reflux oesophagitis changes are most commonly seen in the distal oesophagus.

7 Answer B: Cricoid impression

8   Answer A: Columnar epithelium replacing stratified squamous epithelium

Barrett's is caused by chronic reflux damaging the epithelium and there are numerous associations. It is a pre-malignant condition hence follow-up is indicated.

9   Answer B: A long distal stricture

Common radiological findings in Barrett's oesophagus include: a long stricture in the mid or lower oesophagus, a large deep solitary ulcer (Barrett's ulcer), a fine reticular mucosal pattern, thickened irregular mucosal folds, a fine granular mucosal pattern and distal oesophageal widening.

10   Answer E: Schatzki ring

A Schatzki ring is a symptomatic, narrow-calibre stenotic ring at the gastro-oesophageal junction. It produces a typical episodic solid dysphagia, which is sometimes known as 'steakhouse syndrome'. The short height (typically 2–4mm) and regular, symmetrical appearance help to distinguish it from malignant, peptic and other strictures.

11   Answer B: 2

The number needed to treat (NNT) is a measure of the effectiveness of the drug and is the number of patients who need to be treated to prevent one death (or other adverse outcome). It is defined as the inverse of the absolute risk reduction. In this case the probability of death in the control group is 40/200 and in the treatment group 20/200, hence the absolute risk reduction is 20/200=0.1 and the NNT is 10. The number needed to harm (NNH) is similar and is the inverse of the attributable risk (the risk in the exposed group minus the risk in the non-exposed group).

12   Answer C: Widespread carcinoid metastases

In 111-labelled octreotide study is used to assess for somatostatin receptor positive carcinoid disease and if positive may indicate that the patient's disease is suitable for radiolabelled treatment. Carcinoid syndrome specifically relates to clinical symptoms in the presence of liver or lung metastases but is not a radiological diagnosis. The CT findings are not typical of lymphoma. Paraganglioma is usually assessed with MIBG but does show octreoscan uptake but the radiological findings are not consistent with this diagnosis.

13   Answer D: Gastric volvulus

Gastric volvulus, although rare, is more common in the elderly population. It may result from twisting in the longitudinal, transverse or mesenteric axis. The dilated stomach usually contains a long fluid level and is displaced upwards and to the left, causing a raised left hemidiaphragm.

14   Answer A: Gastric duplication cyst

This two-layered appearance is classic of gastric duplication cyst. Sixty-five per cent are in the region of the greater curvature. Most present in infancy with 75% being detected before the age of 12 years.

15 Answer B: Hampton's line

Benign features	Malignant features
Protrudes beyond stomach	No protrusion
Deep	Shallow
Round/oval	Irregular shape
Symmetrical	Asymmetrical
Smooth collar	No collar
Hampton's line present	Hampton's line absent
Smooth even folds	Irregular nodular folds
No adjacent masses/nodules	Adjacent nodules
Heals completely	Rarely completely heals

16 Answer B: Thickened folds in the proximal stomach

This is hypertrophic gastritis and may present with epigastric pain, achlorydia, and protein loss. There are thickened gastric folds mainly in the proximal stomach and greater curve. Unlike in a malignant process the stomach wall does not become rigid, but endoscopy and biopsy are usually necessary for diagnosis.

17 Answer C: Hyperplastic polyps

Hyperplastic polyps occur mainly in the body and fundus of the stomach but also randomly throughout the stomach. They normally measure under 1 cm in size, but rarely be 3–10 cm. This type makes up 80–90% of gastric polyps.

18 Answer E: Erosive gastritis

Erosive (haemorrhagic) gastritis is associated with peptic disease, infection and Crohn's disease. Non-steroidal anti-inflammatory drugs are a common underlying cause, which may have been used to treat his back pain. Contrast studies may show complete or incomplete erosions. Complete erosions show a spot of barium surrounded by a radiolucent ring of oedema (target lesion). Incomplete erosions show dots and linear streaks of barium without associated oedema.

19 Answer D: Greater curvature located cranially

Features	Organoaxial volvulus	Mesenteroaxial volvulus
Mechanism	Rotation around long axis of stomach	Rotation around short axis
Appearance	Greater curvature rotated cranially – 'upside-down' stomach	Fundus is caudal to antrum

(continued)

Features	Organoaxial volvulus	Mesenteroaxial volvulus
Predisposed	Adults with large hiatal hernia	Large portions of stomach above diaphragm (e.g. traumatic diaphragmatic rupture in children)
Complications	Rare	Common (obstruction, ischaemia)

20 Answer A: Cystic fibrosis

Cystic fibrosis affects the gastrointestinal tract in the majority of patients and manifestations include: meconium plugging, meconium ileus, distal intestinal obstruction, gastro-oesophageal reflux, thickened duodenal folds, small bowel dilatation, colonic stricturing, microcolon and pneumatosis intestinalis.

21 Answer B: Leiomyoma

Leiomyoma are the most common benign small bowel tumours and are responsible for half of cases of small bowel haemorrhage. Their usual presentation is with bleeding from the ulcerated tumour surface in the small bowel. Carcinoma is rare in the small bowel. Carcinoids represent 1.5% of all GI neoplasms and most commonly occur in the appendix. Ultrasound may show a broad-based intraluminal mass in the early stages. The small bowel is involved in 30% of lymphoma and usually a mass, either circumferential or extending along the bowel, is visible.

22 Answer A: Linear ulcers on mesenteric border

Linear ulcers on the mesenteric border are nearly pathognomonic of Crohn's disease. Ulcers are most commonly multiple in inflammatory bowel disease. Double tracking ulcers are usually seen in the colon in the context of ulcerative colitis.

23 Answer E: Peutz-Jeghers syndrome

Peutz-Jeghers is a relatively rare autosomal-dominant condition that is characterised by the presence of gastrointestinal polyps and mucocutaneous pigmentation. The polyps are mainly seen in the small bowel and are classically broad based. In the presence of abdominal pain intussusception occurs in up to 47%.

24 Answer B: Hydrostatic reduction at 120 mmHg

A rule of threes usually applies: maximum three attempts for three minutes, allowing three minutes between attempts. The pressure should be approximately 120 mmHg. (The colonic bursting pressure is approximately 200 mmHg.)

25 Answer B: Appendix

Commonest sites are appendix (>60%) and small bowel 20% (distal 2 feet of ileum). They are rare in the rectum and stomach and virtually never occur in the oesophagus.

26 Answer C: Rectal involvement

Rectal involvement is commoner in ulcerative colitis (UC) (95%) than Crohn's (50%).

27 Answer B: Intussusception

There are many causes of false positive Tc-99m pertechnetate studies which include: ectopic gastric mucosa, enteric duplication, Barrett's oesophagus, arteriovenous malformations, haemangiomata, hypervascular tumour, aneurysm, duodenal ulcer, ulcerative colitis, Crohn's disease, appendicitis, intussusception, bowel obstruction and urinary tract obstruction. Ileal rotation, haemorrhage and rapid bowel transit are causes of a false negative study.

28 Answer A: Angiodysplasia of the colon

Angiodysplasia of the colon is the most common vascular malformation of the GI tract and is due to vascular ectasia rather than a true arteriovenous malformation (AVM). It is caused by age-related degenerative dilatation and is associated with aortic stenosis in 20%. It is most commonly seen in the caecum/ascending colon.

29 Answer C: Lynch II

Lynch is otherwise known as hereditary nonpolyposis colorectal cancer syndrome. The Amsterdam criteria of this syndrome are based on relatives who have been diagnosed with colorectal cancer. (Three or more family members of whom two are first-degree relatives of the third, family members in two or more generations, one family member diagnosed <50 years old.) It is present in 5–10% of individuals with colon cancer. Lynch I has no association with extracolonic malignancies. Lynch II is associated with other malignancies including transitional cell carcinoma of the ureter and renal pelvis.

30 Answer D: Pulmonary disease

There are over 60 causative factors for pneumatosis intestinalis. However, there are four main mechanisms by which they occur: bowel necrosis/gangrene, mucosal disruption, increased mucosal permeability and pulmonary disease. As a general rule pneumatosis of the colon is likely to be clinically insignificant and the extent of the pneumatosis is inversely related to the severity of the disease. A well man is unlikely to have ischaemic bowel and with a significant smoking history and probable symptomatic lung disease then pulmonary disease is the most likely cause. He has no good history for the other two mechanisms. Gas can be seen in the mesenteric and portal veins with pulmonary disease.

31 Answer B: Free intra-abdominal air

In necrotising enterocolitis, pneumatosis intestinalis is seen in 80%. Gas in the portal vein can be seen, is frequently transient and does not imply a terrible outcome as it would in adults. Pneumoperitoneum is a poor prognostic factor and usually requires immediate surgery.

32 Answer C: *Cytomegalovirus* (CMV)

CMV is the commonest cause of life-threatening opportunistic infection in AIDS patients and accounts for 13% of all gastrointestinal disease in this population.

33 Answer D: Caecal volvulus

Caecal volvulus accounts for 40% of all colonic volvuluses and is associated with malrotation and a long mesentery giving poor fixation of the right colon (10–25% of the population). If caecal distension greater than 10–12 cm occurs, there is an increased risk of perforation or bowel infarction.

34 Answer B: Ileocaecal

Crohn's disease is the third commonest cause of fistula after iatrogenic and diverticular fistulae. Enterocolic are most often between ileum and caecum; other fistula may occur: enterocutaneous (8–21%), rectum to skin or vagina, peri-anal fistulae and sinus tracts.

35 Answer A: Ill-defined margins

	True polyp	Pseudopolyp
Size	Uniform in size	Uniform in size
Form	Round, stalked, sessile	Y-shaped, filiform, irregular
Margins	Well-delineated	Fuzzy (inflammation)
Colonic haustra	Preserved	Distorted (inflammation)

36 Answer E: Sigmoid volvulus

Sigmoid volvulus is common in elderly and psychiatric patients. The typical plain radiograph appearance is of a dilated loop of sigmoid with a distinct midline crease – the 'coffee-bean' sign. Twisting of the mesentery is seen on CT.

37 Answer A: Ultrasound of the liver with Doppler

Doppler ultrasound is a reliable, non-invasive method in assessing shunt patency.

Feldstein VA, Patel MD, LaBerge JM, *et al*. Transjugular intrahepatic porto-systemic shunts: accuracy of Doppler US in determination of patency and detection of stenoses. *Radiology*. 1996; **201**(1): 141–7.

38 Answer C: Chronic Budd-Chiari syndrome

In acute Budd-Chiari syndrome the caudate lobe does not hypertrophy as it does in the chronic form (as it has separate drainage directly into the IVC). There are various causes of Budd-Chiari syndrome; 66% are idiopathic.

39 Answer C: Central scar

40 Answer A: Ascitic fluid

The Child-Pugh score is derived from bilirubin and albumin levels, prothrombin time, hepatic encephalopathy and presence ascites.

41 Answer B: Colorectal

Colorectal > Gastric > Pancreatic > Breast > Lung

42 Answer B: *Entamoeba histolytica*

Amoebic abscesses typically present as a large solitary lesion in the right lobe of the liver. The contents have been described as 'anchovy paste' or 'chocolate sauce'.

43 Answer E: Budd-Chiari syndrome

Occlusion of the hepatic veins/IVC, often due to thrombosis in hypercoagulable states such as pregnancy. Hepatosplenomegaly, with caudate hypertrophy, are early sonographic signs with non-visualisation of the hepatic veins in 75%. Symptoms also include right heart failure and pulmonary oligaemia.

44 Answer C: Beta-thalassaemia

All the options are causes of hepatosplenomegaly. Beta-thalassaemia is more common in the Mediterranean population and can cause microcytic anaemia and abnormal liver function. Affected patients are at increased risk of developing gallstones.

45 Answer C: 25–50% of the surface area

There are five grades of splenic injury depending on surface area involved, depth of laceration and vascular involvement.

46 Answer A: Diffuse/focal low signal on T1 and T2

Splenic angiosarcoma is rare with less than 100 reported cases. It usually presents in patients aged 50–60 years and MRI shows diffuse or focal areas of low signal on T1 and T2 due to haemorrhage, which results in iron deposition.

47 Answer B: Melanoma

Metastases account for 7% of solid splenic tumours. Melanoma accounts for 6–34%.

48 Answer D: Lymphoma

The differential diagnosis for a focal low-density splenic lesion includes: lymphoma, metastases, haemangioma and abscess. In this case the concurrent lymphadenopathy and normal septic markers suggest lymphoma.

49 Answer B: Gut malrotation

Polysplenia (bilateral left-sidedness) typically presents in infancy and is associated with a variety of congenital cardiac, gastrointestinal, genito-urinary and skeletal abnormalities. Malrotation is present in 80%.

50 Answer A: Carcinoma of the gallbladder

An irregular focal area of wall thickening is suggestive of gallbladder carcinoma.

Risk factors include increased body mass, female gender, post-menopausal status and cigarette smoking. In up to 90% of gallbladder carcinomas cholelithiasis is present.

51 Answer B: 5–15%

Sludge on ultrasound is seen as dependent echoes that do not cause shadowing. Common causes are chronic fasting, total parental nutrition, critical illness, ceftriaxone therapy and pregnancy. Spontaneous resolution occurs in 50% of patients and 5–15% will go on to develop gallstones.

52 Answer E: Percutaneous cholecystostomy

Percutaneous cholecystostomy can often be performed in poor surgical candidates or acutely unwell patients.

53 Answer A: Infiltration of liver

Carcinoma of the gallbladder most commonly spreads by direct extension into the liver. Lymphatic spread and peritoneal seeding are also common. Neural spread tends to be associated with more aggressive tumours. Haematogenous spread is relatively rare.

54 Answer B: Dilatation of the distal intramural portion of the common bile duct that protrudes in the duodenum

A choledochocele is cystic dilatation of the distal/intramural duodenal portion of the common bile duct with herniation of the duct into the duodenum.

55 Answer C: *Escherichia coli*

Gram-negative enteric bacteria are the usual causative agent in ascending cholangitis, the commonest being *E. coli*.

56 Answer C: Choledochal cyst

Choledochal cysts are formed by cystic dilatation of the intra- or extrahepatic biliary ducts. The diagnosis is established at cholangiography. Caroli's disease affects only the intrahepatic ducts.

57 Answer D: Caroli's disease

The best diagnostic clue is the 'central dot' sign – strongly enhancing central tiny dots and the presence of renal tubular ectasia. Patients often present in their second to third decade with recurrent cholangitis. ERCP, MRCP and technetium colloid sulphur are most helpful.

58 Answer C: Lymphatic spread to cystic lymph nodes

Lymphatic spread to cystic nodes 32%, infiltration of liver 23%, lymphatic spread to coeliac nodes 16%, peritoneal seeding 9%, haematogenous spread is rare.

59 Answer B: Duodenum

60 Answer D: Gallstone ileus

61 Answer D: Lymphoma

This is a 'soft' tumour, which does not usually obstruct ducts.

62 Answer E: Pancreatic islet cell tumour

Pancreatic islet cell tumours are often small (<2 cm) and multiple and can often be difficult to detect. They are usually iso-attenuating on unenhanced CT but show avid enhancement in arterial phase. Metastases to the liver occur in 60–90% of cases with or without lymph node involvement and are often hypervascular. The average time from onset of symptoms to diagnosis is 2.7 years.

63 Answer E: Whipple's procedure with normal post-operative appearances

A standard Whipple's procedure is a pancreaticoduodenectomy. There are three main anastomoses: a gastrojejunostomy, a choledochojejunostomy and a pancreaticojejunostomy.

64 Answer B: Hereditary pancreatitis

Hereditary pancreatitis is inherited in an autosomal dominant fashion. It is the most common cause of large spherical pancreatitic calcifications in childhood and causes repeat episodes of pancreatitis. Twenty to forty per cent develop pancreatitic carcinoma and pseudocyst formation is seen in 50%.

65 Answer D: Splenic artery

Post-inflammatory pseudoaneurysms can rupture into pre-existing pseudocysts and are caused by digestion of the arterial wall by released enzymes. This occurs in up to 10% of patients with severe pancreatitis. The splenic artery is the most common site and there is significant (approximately 35%) mortality if they rupture.

66 Answer E: Ultrasound of the abdomen

In an overweight middle-aged female the most common cause of acute pancreatitis is gallstone disease. This is even more likely in the context of abnormal liver function tests. A gallstone-causing obstruction in the common bile duct should be excluded with ultrasound as this would probably require intervention. CT is mainly indicated in the context of assessment of complications.

67 Answer B: Grade II injury
Grade I: Minor contusion/haematoma, capsule and major duct intact
Grade II: Parenchymal injury without major duct injury
Grade III: Major ductal injury
Grade IV: Severe crush injury

68 Answer C: Hypovascularity

Features	Serous microcystic adenoma (benign)	Mucinous cystic neoplasm (malignant potential)
Number of cysts	>6	<6
Size of individual cysts	<20 mm	>20 mm
Calcification	40%: amorphous, starbursts	20%: rim calcification
Enhancement	Hypervascular	Hypovascular
Cyst content (aspiration)	Glycogen	Mucin
Other features	Central scar (15%)	Peripheral enhancement
		Spread: local. LN, liver
Demographics	Older patients (>60 years)	Younger patients (40–60 years)
Location	70% in head of pancreas	95% in body or tail of pancreas

69 Answer A: Dilatation of pancreatic duct

Only 8–15% of pancreatic adenocarcinomas are resectable at the time of presentation. Resectable tumours are typically isolated pancreatic masses with or without dilatation of the pancreatic or biliary ducts. Features of irresectable tumours include: extension of tumour beyond the margins of the pancreas, tumour invasion of adjacent organs, enlarged regional lymph nodes and encasement of peripancreatic arteries and veins.

70 Answer B: Deep fissures and large shallow linear ulcers with elevated margins

In primary intestinal tuberculosis the classical presentation is with weight loss and abdominal pain and the tuberculin skin test is negative in most patients. The ulcerative form is the most common manifestation and disease is usually seen in the ileocaecal area. Deep fissures and large shallow linear/stellate ulcers with elevated margins are characteristic.

Gastrointestinal and hepatobiliary radiology

PAPER 3: ANSWERS AND EXPLANATIONS

1 Answer A: Oesophageal varices

2 Answer E: 7

3 Answer C: Thicker valvulae conniventes

Jejunum	Ileum
3–3.5 cm diameter	2.5 cm diameter
Thicker valvulae conniventes	Thinner valvulae conniventes
1–2 arterial arcades	3–4 arterial arcades
Thicker walls	Thinner walls
Fewer, larger Peyer's patches	More Peyer's patches

4 Answer C: Polypoid protuberance arising near cardia

This is the most common appearance of an inflammatory polyp.

5 Answer B: Chagas disease

Chagas disease characteristically involves diffuse oesophageal dilatation, mega-colon and cardiomegaly.

6 Answer A: Achalasia

In achalasia the lower oesophageal sphincter fails to relax due to Wallerian degeneration of Auerbach's plexus. Relaxation only occurs when hydrostatic pressure exceeds that of the sphincter. There are three forms: (1) primary (idiopathic) or (2) secondary due to metastases or invasion of adenocarcinoma of the cardia, or (3) infectious (e.g., Chagas disease). The primary form classically occurs in 20–30 year olds, with dysphagia to both solids and liquids with weight loss. Two diagnostic criteria are absent primary and secondary waves, and failure of the lower oesophageal sphincter to relax. Other features are tertiary contractions, oesophageal dilatation and a bird's beak appearance. There may be an air fluid level on plain films. Complications include recurrent aspiration and pneumonia in 10%, and an increased incidence of oesophageal malignancy. It is important to distinguish idiopathic achalasia from malignancy and oesophageal spasm.

7   Answer D: Oesophageal leiomyoma

Leiomyomas are the commonest benign oesophageal neoplasm. They arise in smooth muscle and are therefore normally intramural. They are commoner in men and in the third to fifth decades. Most are asymptomatic and found incidentally, but they can cause dysphagia and pain.

8   Answer B: CMV oesophagitis

The finding of a large solitary oesophageal ulcer in an HIV positive patient is most likely to represent either CMV oesophagitis or HIV oesophagitis. These two conditions are radiologically indistinguishable.

9   Answer B: Lymphoma

The presence of a polypoidal mass associated with mediastinal lymphadenopathy is most suggestive of oesophageal lymphoma. The oesophagus is the least common site of gastrointestinal lymphoma. More common sites include the stomach, small bowel and colon.

10   Answer D: Origin at Killian's dehiscence

Zenker's diverticulum originates in the midline of the posterior oesophageal wall at a point known as Killian's dehiscence (above cricopharyngeus). It bulges during swallowing. Killian-Jamieson diverticula originate below cricopharyngeus.

11   Answer D: N1 M1b

Assuming the primary shows uptake then PET-CT allows accurate assessment of nodal disease particularly if they are normal by size criteria. The presence of a positive coeliac axis node in this patient upstages him to N1, M1b and makes him unsuitable for curative surgery. Tumour staging is assessed by endorectal ultrasonography (EUS).

12   Answer C: Radionuclide HIDA scan

White cell labelled radionuclide scans are used for the investigation of low-grade infection when no abnormality is seen on conventional imaging. MRCP is useful for imaging the biliary tree for strictures and stones but the length of time to acquire images and lack of functional imaging makes it unsuitable to diagnose a biloma. Although a collection on CT in the correct clinical setting will usually indicate a biloma a HIDA scan will demonstrate biliary excretion of Tc labelled IDA at 30 minutes and activity in the right paracolic space/peritoneum indicates a bile leak.

13   Answer B: Duodenal atresia

Duodenal atresia is the most common cause of congenital duodenal obstruction.

Twenty-five per cent of neonates with atresia have Down syndrome as in this case.

14 Answer C: Peptic ulcer disease

In gastric outlet obstruction caused by inflammatory narrowing 60–65% is caused by peptic ulcer disease. This is particularly likely in a patient with a history of symptoms probably related to peptic ulcer disease.

15 Answer C: Zollinger-Ellison syndrome

Zollinger-Ellison syndrome is secondary to a functional pancreatic islet cell tumour producing gastrin. It causes gastric hypersecretion, which leads to multiple ulcers and a diffuse inflammatory response accounting for the thickened folds.

16 Answer B: Blind loop syndrome

This occurs following a Billroth II procedure when the afferent loop intermittently partially obstructs and overdistends. Typical features on a contrast examination would be preferential emptying of the stomach into the proximal loop, stasis and regurgitation.

17 Answer E: Submucosal metastases

The commonest cause of 'bull's-eye' lesions in the stomach is submucosal metastases and of these the commonest primary tumour is malignant melanoma. Other causes of gastric 'bull's-eye' lesions include: leiomyoma, pancreatic rest and neurofibroma.

18 Answer E: Submucosal umbilicated mass

Pancreatic rests (ectopic pancreas) typically occur in the greater curvature, pylorus, duodenal bulb or proximal jejunum. They manifest as submucosal nodules between 1 and 5 cm in size. Central umbilication is often present, representing the orifice of the filiform duct.

19 Answer A: Carman's (meniscus) sign

Radiological signs of a malignant ulcer include: thick irregular mucosal folds, projection of ulcer within luminal surface, Carman's (meniscus) sign, eccentric location of ulcer in tumour mound, a thick nodular irregular collar and limited gastric distensibility and peristalsis.

20 Answer B: Duodenum

Ninety-five per cent of intestinal trauma occurs in the duodenum and proximal jejunum. The remaining 5% occurs in the colon. Blunt intestinal trauma at other sites is rare.

21 Answer E: Carcinoid of small bowel with a concurrent colorectal malignancy

Carcinoid tumours are the most common primary tumour of the small bowel and appendix. One-third of carcinoids are seen in the small bowel and 91% of these are in the ileum. They are classically submucosal vascular lesions and are associated with low-density lymphadenopathy due to necrosis. Approximately 30% have a second primary malignancy of the gastrointestinal tract.

22 Answer A: Right paraduodenal hernia

A right paraduodenal hernia is the most common internal hernia and classically displaces the inferior mesenteric vein.

23 Answer C: Carcinoid tumour

This is a description of retractile mesenteritis and is associated with all the listed conditions. However, the enhancing submucosal lesion in the ileum is a classic appearance and site of a carcinoid tumour.

24 Answer A: Crohn's disease

The age of presentation of Crohn's disease is typically 15–30 years with an equal sex distribution. The symptoms are often vague and may be present for some time before the diagnosis is made. It can affect any part of the GI tract from the mouth to the anus and can skip segments.

25 Answer C: Behcet's syndrome

This is a chronic granulomatous inflammatory disease of unknown aetiology. The natural course is relapsing and there is a triad of aphthous stomatitis, genital ulcers and ocular inflammation. Age of onset is the third decade and it affects twice as many males as females.

26 Answer C: Mesenteric mass

27 Answer E: Systemic mastocytosis

Causes of tiny small bowel nodules include: nodular lymphoid hyperplasia, lymphoma, amyloidosis, Whipple disease, *Mycobacterium avium-intracellulare*, lymphangiectasia and systemic mastocytosis.

28 Answer A: MR fistulography

29 Answer B: The inferior mesenteric artery is evaluated before the superior mesenteric artery

The inferior mesenteric artery is usually evaluated first as once the patient's bladder begins to fill with contrast it may become more difficult to evaluate this area. The celiac axis is not routinely assessed when investigating lower gastrointestinal bleeding.

30 Answer D: T3 N1 M0

31 Answer C: Ischaemic colitis

The commonest cause of acute ischaemic bowel is an occlusive superior mesenteric artery (SMA) embolus – in more than 50% of cases. Other causes are non-occlusive thrombus, SMA dissection and venous occlusion.

32 Answer B: Angiodysplasia

This is due to age-related degeneration and dilatation of the submucosal vessels in the bowel wall and is the commonest vascular lesion of the GI tract. The caecum and ascending colon are most commonly affected followed by the descending and sigmoid colon. Less frequently, the small bowel may also be affected.

33 Answer E: Sigmoid volvulus

This is commoner in the elderly and institutionalised populations. Varying degrees of torsion can occur, the commonest being through 360 degrees.

34 Answer B: <5 mm

The normal pre-sacral space in adults in 95% of cases is <5 mm and abnormal is >10 mm.

35 Answer B: Lobulation

Feature	Benign polyp	Malignant polyp
Size	<1 cm	>2 cm
Stalk	Present (pedunculated, thin)	Absent (sessile)
Contour	Smooth	Irregular, lobulated
Number	Single	Multiple
Underlying colonic wall	Smooth	Indented, retracted

36 Answer B: Right hemicolon

37 Answer A: Hypointense T1 and hyperintense T2

38 Answer C: Cardiac failure

39 Answer C: Increased periportal attenuation

40 Answer A: Adenoma

Most focal liver lesions are hypointense on T1WI. Exceptions to this rule include: adenoma, fatty lesions, blood, proteinaceous material, melanoma metastases and contrast agents.

41 Answer C: MRI

Sensitivity for detection of liver metastases: MR > CECT > FDG PET-CT.

42 Answer B: Hepatic artery

Unlike pyogenic and amoebic infections, which usually enter the liver via the biliary ducts or portal vein, fungal infections typically enter via the hepatic artery.

43 Answer D: Budd-Chiari syndrome

44 Answer C: Splenic infarct secondary to embolic phenomenon

Splenic infarction commonly presents with left upper quadrant pain and fever in the acute setting. An elevated ESR and leucocytosis are often seen. A wedge-shaped infarct will be more ill defined acutely on ultrasound secondary to oedema and inflammation. The most common cause of infarct is due to embolic phenomenon, particularly in an arteriopath.

45 Answer B: 40–60 HU

Unenhanced CT spleen approximately 40–60 HU, and 5–10 HU less than liver.

46 Answer B: Bacterial endocarditis

Splenic infarcts can be either peripheral and wedge shaped, or rounded irregularly shaped and randomly distributed. Fifty per cent of the cardiovascular-caused splenic infarcts are due to bacterial endocarditis.

47 Answer B: Granulomas

There are numerous causes of splenic calcifications; the morphology and distribution varies according to aetiology. The commonest cause of disseminated splenic calcification is granulomatous disease, such as histoplasmosis, TB and brucellosis.

48 Answer D: Sarcoidosis

Erythema nodosum is the most common presentation of sarcoid (30%). Hepatobiliary manifestations of sarcoid include: hepatomegaly, splenomegaly, nodular lesions in the liver and spleen, lymphadenopathy and pancreatic mass.

A general differential diagnosis for splenomegaly includes:

- huge spleen: chronic myeloid leukaemia, myelofibrosis, malaria, Kala-azar, Gaucher's disease, lymphoma
- moderately enlarged spleen: all of the above plus storage diseases, haemolytic anaemias, portal hypertension and leukaemias
- slightly enlarged spleen: all of the above plus infections, sarcoidosis, amyloidosis, rheumatoid arthritis and systemic lupus erythematosus.

49 Answer A: Arc-like hyperechogenic areas outlining the gallbladder wall

Intramural gas can occur with any severe cholecystitis that causes gross inflammation and compromises the gallbladder wall. Arc-like echoes that outline the gallbladder wall represents gas within the gallbladder itself, which occurs in emphysematous cholecystitis and not simple acute cholecystitis. Emphysematous cholecystitis is associated with calculous and is more prevalent in diabetics. Complications include gallbladder gangrene and perforation. The halo sign is a three-layered configuration of the gallbladder wall with a lucent middle layer, which represents oedema and is a common observation in acute cholecystitis.

50 Answer B: Non-shadowing and mobile

	Common cause	Less common
Shadowing, mobile	Stones	Nil
Non-shadowing, mobile	Sludge	Small stones (<3 mm)
Non-shadowing, non-mobile	Polyps	Sludge

51 Answer E: Gallbladder perforation

Gallbladder perforation occurs in 5–10% of patients with acute cholecystitis. Localised disruption of the gallbladder wall is seen on ultrasound in less than 40% of cases and CT in 80%.

52 Answer B: *Clostridium perfringens*

Clostridium perfringens is the most common cause of emphysematous cholecystitis. There is an approximately 15% mortality.

53 Answer B: Non-visualisation of the gallbladder by four hours

(Ninety-nine per cent specific.)

54 Answer B: Ampullary tumour

Ampullary tumours have an association with FAP syndrome. The tumour is often inconspicuous due to its small size. Peri-ampullary tumours are usually larger lesions with significant intraduodenal extension.

55 Answer A: Primary sclerosing cholangitis (PSC)

PSC is more common in males by approx 2:1. Usually presents by 45 years.

56 Answer E: Fistulation between the gallbladder and common hepatic duct

In Mirizzi's syndrome a gallstone impacts in the gallbladder neck or cystic duct and causes extrinsic compression of the common hepatic duct. It is frequently associated with the formation of a fistula between the gallbladder and common hepatic duct.

57 Answer D: *Cytomegalovirus*

CMV and *cryptococcus* are the most common opportunistic infective organisms. HIV can also cause cholangitis but is not an opportunistic infection.

58 Answer C: Intrahepatic cholangiocarcinoma

There is a predilection for the right lobe and this accounts for around 10% of all cholangiocarcinomas. Up to 20% are resectable. The peripheral washout sign and delayed enhancement on CT are suggestive.

59 Answer E: Choledochal cyst

Communication to common hepatic/intrahepatic duct is vital for diagnosis.

HIDA uptake is variable, but a positive result shows a photopenic area that fills in within 60 minutes, with a paucity of contrast in the small bowel.

60 Answer C: Intrahepatic cholangiocarcinoma

Increased risk in inflammatory bowel disease (by 10×) particularly ulcerative colitis and primary sclerosing cholangitis (PSC) with a latent period of approximately 15 years. Right lobar predilection. Poor prognosis.

61 Answer D: Congenital tracheobiliary fistula

The finding of pneumobilia is key to thinking of the diagnosis.

62 Answer A: Haemorrhagic pancreatitis

The hyperdense areas in the gland represent acute haemorrhage. All the other options, except calcification, produce areas of low attenuation and calcification would be greater than 50–70 HU.

63 Answer D: Non-compressible tubular structure >6 mm thick

Ultrasound features of appendicitis are total thickness >6 mm, non-compressibility, wall thickness >3 mm and a shadowing appendicolith.

64 Answer C: Insulinoma

MEN I syndrome is strongly associated with pancreatic islet cell tumours. Insulinomas are more likely to be multiple in MEN I and are usually hypointense on T1 and hyperintense on T2. Tumours over 2 cm show ring enhancement.

65 Answer C: Pancreatic contusion

The area of low attenuation with the gland is consistent with a parenchymal contusion. If haemorrhage was present his would probably be of increased attenuation.

66 Answer D: Ultrasound abdomen

67 Answer B: Hyperparathyroidism

Pancreatitis complicates 10% of hyperparathyroidism. The pattern of pancreatic calcification is indistinguishable from alcoholic pancreatitis, but the presence of renal tract calcification is highly suggestive of hyperparathyroidism.

68 Answer A: Chronic pancreatitis

In chronic pancreatitis, repeated episodes of mild or subclinical pancreatitis lead to irreversible destruction of the parenchyma. The gland is often small and atrophic, but focal enlargement is present in 40%. Parenchymal calcification, fatty replacement and fibrosis are also features.

69 Answer E: Unseen ovarian tumour

The three classical causes of high-density ascites are tuberculosis, ovarian tumour and appendiceal tumour, which produce particularly proteinaceous fluid. Other exudates may also cause ascites of higher density: Meigs syndrome is an exudative process, but no pleural effusion was present. A simple transudate is likely to be of lower attenuation, for example Budd-Chiari syndrome.

70 Answer C: Mastocytosis

Mastocytosis is a systemic disease where there is mast cell proliferation. Over 50% present before six months old. Urticaria pigmentosa is seen in up to 90% and disease is seen in the skeletal, reticuloendothelial and abdominal systems.

Bibliography

GENERAL REFERENCE TEXTS

Adam A, Dixon A, editors. *Grainger & Allison's Diagnostic Radiology: a textbook of medical imaging*. 5th ed. London: Churchill Livingstone; 2007.

Brandt WE, Helms CA. *Fundamentals of Diagnostic Radiology*. 3rd ed. Philadelphia, PA: Lippincott, Williams & Wilkins; 2007.

Chapman S, Nakielny R. *Aids to Radiological Differential Diagnosis*. 4th ed. Philadelphia, PA: Saunders; 2003.

Dahnert W. *Radiology Review Manual*. 6th ed. Philadelphia, PA: Lippincott, Williams & Wilkins; 2007.

Federle M, editor. *Diagnostic Imaging: abdomen*. Salt Lake City, UT: Amirsys; 2004.

Husband JE, Reznek RH, editors. *Imaging in Oncology*. London: Taylor and Francis; 2004.

Middleton WD, Kurtz AB, Hertzberg BS. *Ultrasound: the requisites*. 2nd ed. St Louis, MO: Mosby; 2003.

Semelka RC, editor. *Abdominal-Pelvic MRI*. New York, NY: Wiley-Liss Inc; 2002.

Webb R, Brandt W, Major NM. *Fundamentals of Body CT*. 3rd ed. Philadelphia, PA: Saunders; 2006.

Weissleder R, Wittenberg M, Harisinghani M. *Primer of Diagnostic Imaging*. 3rd ed. St Louis, MO: Mosby; 2003.

ANAPHYLAXIS

Resuscitation Council (UK). *Guidelines on Emergency Treatment of Anaphylactic Reactions*. London: Resuscitation Council (UK); 2008. Available at: www.resus.org.uk (accessed 15 February 2009).

CONTRAST MEDIA

The European Society of Urogenital Radiology. *ESUR Guidelines on Contrast Media, version 6.0*. The European Society of Urogenital Radiology; 2007. Available at: www.esur.org (accessed 15 February 2009).

INTERVENTION

Kessel D, Robertson I. *Interventional Radiology: a survival guide*. 2nd ed. London: Churchill Livingstone; 2005.

CARDIOTHORACIC RADIOLOGY

Webb WR, Higgins CB. *Thoracic Imaging: pulmonary and cardiovascular radiology*. Philadelphia, PA: Lippincott, Williams & Wilkins; 2004.

MUSCULOSKELETAL RADIOLOGY AND TRAUMA

Raby N. *Accident and Emergency Radiology: a survival guide*. 2nd ed. Philadelphia, PA: Saunders; 2005.

GASTROINTESTINAL RADIOLOGY

Gore RM, Levine MS. *Textbook of Gastrointestinal Radiology*. 3rd ed. Philadelphia, PA: Saunders; 2007.

PAEDIATRIC RADIOLOGY

Burton EM, Brody AS. *Essentials of Pediatric Radiology*. New York, NY: Thieme; 1999.

Chen H. *Atlas of Genetic Diagnosis and Counselling*. Totowa, NJ: Humana Press; 2005.

Kim D, Betz RR, editors. *Surgery of the Pediatric Spine*. New York, NY: Thieme; 2008.

Siegel MJ, Coley B, editors. *Pediatric Imaging*. Philadelphia, PA: Lippincott, Williams & Wilkins; 2005.

Staheli LT. *Fundamentals of Pediatric Orthopedics*. Philadelphia, PA: Lippincott, Williams & Wilkins; 2003.

Index

Note: Questions and answers are given in the following format Q/A.